Disclaimer

We are not a medical doctor nor is this intended to give you health advice. It is not a substitute for professional medical advice, diagnosis or treatment. Always seek the advice of your physician or other qualified health provider with any questions you may have regarding a medical condition.

About the Author

Kyle Newell is the CEO and founder of Newell Strength, located in Central New Jersey.

Kyle has been one of the most 'outside the box' thinkers in the industry of fitness and nutrition since he first entered the field 20 years ago. The road to creating the Panda Diet was paved with hard knocks, experience on the bodybuilding stage, mentoring and coaching from some of the top experts in the world including Scott Abel and John 'Mountain Dog' Meadows.

More importantly, Kyle lives a life dedicated to his wonderful wife, Devon, aka Suzy Homemaker, their 2 sons, Braxton (Munchie), Colt (Tank) and baby daughter, Emma (the Little Warrior). Not to mention two labs, Dax and Mateena.

Some of Kyle's interests are reading, Halloween (Halloween 1 is his absolute favorite movie) and researching the paranormal—in particular, Bigfoot.

Yes, he is quite weird, but that's what you get with a thought leader.

THE PANDA DIET

An Unconventional Approach to Eating
For More Energy and Lasting Weight Loss

Kyle Newell, MS
Founder of Newell Strength

PAGE RESERVED FOR PUBLISHER INFORMATION

"To my wife Devon, thank you for all your support and always pushing me to go for my dreams and to more importantly, to share my dreams and vision with the world, no matter how outside the box they are. And to Brax, Colt and Emma, love you guys and I hope when you are older you'll be proud of this book!"

Contents

Introduction to the Panda Diet Philosophy

If you were to be a fly on the wall right now watching me write this portion of the book, you would notice that I am wearing my panda hat and that I have a corresponding panda tattoo on my wrist.

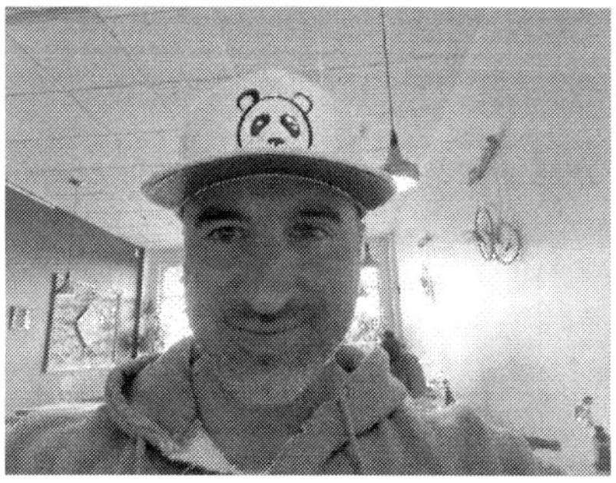

So, how'd this come to be, you ask?

Truth be told, I am a big basketball fan, and one of the players that I have always felt like a kindred spirit to in a lot of ways was Ron Artest. He is only a few years older than I and I loved his tough style of play.

Anyhow, I am not sure how I came to find out that he had an apparel line called the Panda's Friend (which he actually changed his name to for a while). I looked it up and liked what the panda represented so I bought a hat.

And since then, I have made it my own. The physical aspect of the panda is this: it is fierce, yet gentle. People confuse its cuddly appearance with weakness, not realizing that a panda bear could rip a human being to shreds.

Easterners knew that pandas existed, but they just didn't speak of them often. Westerners used to believe that pandas were a fictional beast, much like fire-breathing dragons.

The first one wasn't discovered by a westerner until 1869, and even then, that was just the hide.

Even now, they are scant in numbers, making them a rare creature indeed. On this aspect, I always personally felt the inner drive to be rare; be the one that always practices the golden rule; be the one that lives differently so that I could live and give differently.

As far as diet, pandas eat mainly bamboo, but still have the digestive tracts of a carnivore. This falls in line with my philosophy that we should mainly be eating whole food, plant based diets and the occasional animal protein if we so choose.

Going deeper, the panda represents the opposing duality of life, the yin and yang, the black and the white, the up and the down. In life, I don't believe we should be lukewarm with anything.

In the Bible, Revelation 3:16 says, "Because you are lukewarm, neither hot or cold, I will spit you out."

Being in the gray area or middle of the road will leave you with average results and will never allow you to move the needle towards your greatest life.

When it comes to changing your body, if you follow 99% of people, you will go over the cliff of failure just like them.

Moderation isn't going to cut it nor will willpower. Either go all in, or stay out completely. The Panda Diet works in part because it is so overly simple with its rules.

Just as a vegetarian won't eat a steak if you push it upon them, when you fast, you fast. There is no 'little bit of this, little bit of that.'

We as humans are meant to fast or feast, not graze.

So, fellow panda, be rare; be the trailblazer and embrace the dual nature of life. It's really the only way to live life to the fullest.

What To Expect From This Book

What the Panda 'Diet' Book is Not

- This book is not being written to impress my peers. I do not care if they agree, in fact, I am sure if they do happen to read this, they will vehemently disagree.

- This book is not being loaded up with references and resources. I will cite necessary references at the end of the book.

- This plan is not actually a diet. I only use the term diet because it is familiar to most people. It is a principle that you will be able to use for the rest of your life. Name me one diet that you can stay on for a number of months, let alone the remainder of your life.

- This plan is not based in the idea of having more willpower. That is the main reason that diets fail (Mind Map principle); because they are based in willpower and the human brain will not continuously do something that it doesn't find pleasurable.

- This plan is not going to fit into what you know about diet and food. In fact, it may shatter many of your paradigms and beliefs that the fact fitness experts have led you to believe. You will certainly catch yourself as many of our clients have, trying to apply the old lenses to this philosophy. It will not fit. And I will be sure to remind you of that.

A true expert is one that has mastered the content to such a degree that he or she could teach it to a 2nd grader. Lucky for me, I used to teach K-4 and it helped me to refine my teaching and boil everything down to its simplest form.

Many in the world of fitness and nutrition want to sell you complex solutions because then it creates a dependency on them.

I believe what I have created is the simplest method is existence.

"Complexity is the enemy of execution."
—Tony Robbins

What the Panda 'Diet' Book Is

- This book describes a habits-based approach to losing weight and getting health that completely goes against the grain.

- This book describes my philosophy developed over 20 years of being immersed in fitness and nutrition, and understanding what leads to permanent weight loss, vitality, and supreme energy.

- This book is infused with Mind Mapping principles to make sure that this is not actually a 'diet' in the traditional sense. A typical diet has a defined end date and is something that you can't wait to be done with. That's a BIG part of why a traditional diet doesn't work (it's based on pure willpower).

- This plan is a mindful, Zen-like approach to food and eating. The panda symbolizes a black and white, ying-yang approach to life. A panda bear is gentle looking to the observer but a ferocious, fierce animal when need be. Life is about harmony, a gentle flow of up and down, east and west, enjoyment and discipline. (See the intro for more on this subject.)

Reforming My Understanding of Nutrition

My Introduction to Fasting

In the spring of 2014, the way I viewed dieting and nutrition was forever changed.

You see, at that time, I was getting ready for two upcoming bodybuilding shows that summer.

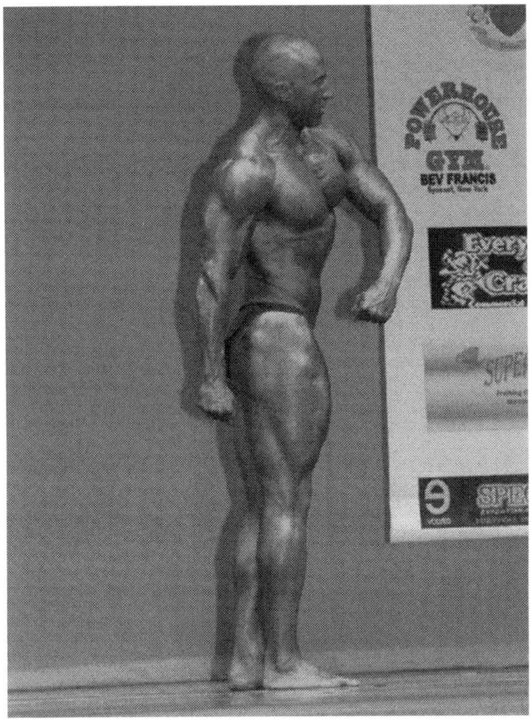

Now, a little back story about me: I had competed in numerous bodybuilding shows during the prior decade and have extensive knowledge and experience with nutrition and diets.

I know that you probably have ZERO thoughts about bodybuilding, but I mention that because it was through those trials and tribulations that I learned the faulty ways of so many of the 'fake fitness experts' (FFE from here on out).

I would do extreme caloric cuts and lose weight—temporarily.

In fact, during each of my competition seasons, I would look ripped and feel terrible. I would also pack on 35-40 pounds after each contest, sometimes even during the first week!!!

If that doesn't tell you that what I was doing was way off course, then nothing will.

Most people don't diet to that extreme, but there are many lessons to learn from the extreme because everything is magnified and easier to observe.

Later on in this book, I will tell you all about the dangers of diets, caloric cuts, and my pendulum theory (yo-yo dieting and weight rebounding).

For now, let's focus on how I came to know fasting and become one of the world's leading experts on the topic.

I was about 8 weeks out from my contests, reading a book about fat loss. In that particular part of that book (by author Lyle McDonald), he was writing about stubborn fat cells and what makes them stubborn.

For women, stubborn fat cells (your alpha receptor cells) are typically located in the glutes and thighs area. For men, they are typically located in the lower abdomen and love handle area.

If you ever put your hand on those areas, you will feel that they are colder to the touch. The reason is that stubborn fat cells lack good blood flow.

This becomes a problem when you look at how fat loss happens. Fat loss is a 3-phase process of mobility, transportation, and utilization. When I talk about mobility, I am speaking of mobilizing fat stores, which is after all, by far the top reason a person would want to 'diet' (not the only reason).

Most people believe that fat loss is a simultaneous process, meaning that if we cut 'X' amount of calories and add 'Y' amount of caloric burn in their workouts, then fat loss and weight loss will magically happen.

If step one, mobility, can only happen under certain conditions, then we can surmise that fat loss and weight loss have a lot more to do with hormonal conditions rather than some arbitrary caloric equation. You will see how this happens in the pages to follow.

• • • • •

Understanding the Fat Loss Process

Step 1:
Your body will only see a need to mobilize fat stores if a hormone known as hormone sensitive lipase is activated. HSL is activated by catecholamine production (adrenaline, nor-adrenaline) and elevated glucagon, which can only be elevated by having low insulin levels. The way you do this is fasting, people have tried to eat low carb, do 'fasted' steady state cardio without much traction.

The theory was along the right lines, but results were short lasting and still are for those that follow this type of approach.

Mobility of the fat cell to use as fuel can only happen if there is adequate blood flow in order to allow us to access that particular fat as an energy source.

When you have poor blood flow, it's not happening.

Well, one of the only proven ways to increase blood flow to the stubborn fat areas is through fasting.

I had no experience with fasting up until I had read that study.

Something clicked in me and the very next day I began my quest of fasting. Keep in mind that I was only fasting for what I thought it would do for me cosmetically at that point, i.e.-to help me drop more body fat before my upcoming contests.

I dove all into the research. I can remember going for a walk with Devon (my wife) and telling her that I had not been as excited about a nutritional concept in forever pretty much. I was on to something.

At that time, from looking back at my notes, I was eating about 1700 calories per day, which is diddly-squat for a guy my size (230 pounds) that was training hard and running a business.

Just to give you an idea, many of my contemporaries with similar builds would be consuming between 3200-4000 calories per day, while getting into contest shape!

But that was what I had come to know as the only way to actually lose body fat from my years of competition and recreational weight loss.

I'd even prescribe the same type of diet to my clients at the time. Cut calories, cut again, and then cut some more. And heck, if you get to a certain deficit and aren't losing any weight then there's not much more else I could do to help you.

It was frustrating for me and frustrating for them.

Allow me to get back on track here with my story though. The very first thing I noticed while eating the exact same quantity of food but cutting back from 4 meals to 2 meals per day was that my hunger was much more manageable.

Whereas following a typical calorie cutting program, my hunger would often get to the point of being intolerable, leading to an otherworldly appetite. And I would fulfill that urge on my 'cheat days', often taking in 15,000 plus calories in the course of 12 hours, something I couldn't even fathom doing now. We will discuss more on that later.

The next thing I noticed was that my digestion was improving. Now, let me be clear, my digestion has always been good, but I used to use a digestive enzyme after some testing found that I was deficient, like 99% of the population.

The reason we are mainly deficient is because stress depletes our main digestive enzyme (hydrochloric acid) and eating too often doesn't give the gut a break, leading to an overworked and inflamed system.

Well, with that particular supplement, you would feel a mild burning sensation if you no longer needed to take it, meaning your 'acid' was back up and running. I was happy to notice that it only took the matter of a month with 16:8 fasting for that to happen.

So, you ask, what the heck is a 16:8? This is the most basic level of fasting in which you have a 16 hour fast every single day, followed by an 8 hour feeding window. It may sound harder than it is, but you have to remember that for much of the 16 hours, you are sleeping. When I first began I would have two feedings per day, which is what I recommend for this type of approach (I outline this later for you).

Lastly, the other thing I noticed in that summer of 2014 was that my body composition was so easy to maintain after the contests. In years prior, I would bloat up so big after the show because of what I was setting my body up for that you wouldn't even recognize me a week later.

I was hooked and have since studied the topic of fasting for thousands of hours, have implemented various fasting protocols with hundreds of clients and have made it one of my life's missions to transform the way people view eating and what's possible when it comes to their health and weight loss.

• • • • •

My Transformed Philosophy on Food and Eating

My personal beliefs have come from a lifetime of experimentation, both on myself and others. Notice that I intentionally called this portion 'food and eating' rather than 'diet'.

This is for a few reasons:

When people hear the very word *diet*, their stress levels usually go up. Your mentality towards the plan you follow will ultimately determine your success, and your mental state has a very large impact on your hormonal profile. As you will soon see, it's the hormones of your body that actually call the shots as to what you get out of an eating program.

The words food and eating are simple. Eating for energy and weight loss should be simple. Too many fake fitness experts want to complicate a subject that should not be complex. They do this either out of their own ignorance, or for reasons of their ego (so that people will dependent on their expertise).

Listen, my life's work has been all about Coaching with a capital C. Coaching is invaluable, when it is entered from a point of view of guidance and wanting to learn and be held accountable. However, the fake fitness experts need to create a dependency from their clients because they fear that if they simplify their teachings, the clients will no longer need them.

With the Panda Diet, you will no longer have to weigh every morsel of food, cut out whole food groups, view carbs as the devil, etc.

You will not have to have guilt about having a 'cheat' meal, nor will you have any more confusion around what you should be doing.

My philosophy is about providing you the teachings and principles that you can keep alive forever, to fit wherever it is in life that you happen to be at that time.

An eating plan must be functional and sustainable to succeed. What this means is that it should be something that you can implement when traveling or when you are out of your home environment and it should be something that you can see yourself doing forever in some form.

Keeping it alive in this program might mean changing your fasting periods throughout the year, depending on goals and circumstance.

My philosophy is based in Mind Mapping. Mind Mapping deals a lot with the human nervous system. To keep it simple, we have two branches that I am concerned with. One of them is known as the sympathetic nervous system (SNS). In this state, you are geared up and ready to go, often in some form of 'fight, flight or freeze'.

Then on the flip side, you have the parasympathetic nervous system (PSNS). In this state you are relaxed, resting, digesting, recovering, and sleeping. With this knowledge, you can see that you would want to be in your PSNS while eating.

A big part of my approach to condensing when you are eating deals with this concept. Most people eat on the run, or eat in 'threatening' environments around people they don't like, or eat while trying to work on their computer or while driving to work.

Most of you that are going to read this are what I would call a busy adult. How many times per day can you realistically sit down to enjoy what you are eating? I would estimate it to be a maximum of two times for most of you. And that's even a stretch to be doing daily.

Here is a simple rule I have about food and eating: if you don't have time to sit down and enjoy the meal, then skip it. You aren't in your correct 'state' to be eating and getting the most out of that meal.

To understand and grasp the principle of fasting, I think we first need to connect the dots on a few of the rampant myths surrounding traditional dieting and diets.

When I am in a consultation with a new client, one of the first things that I want them to understand is that food is a drug.

A drug is something that affects the internal, biochemical and hormonal environment of the body.

Realizing that food is a drug is important because you will then be able to recognize some of the drug like effects food can have on you.

I distinctly remember when I first started with longer form fasting, 48 hours plus, when I would catch myself thinking about food, but not being physically hungry. It would make me question where those thoughts were coming from.

The second thing that I want people to realize is that the main reason we store body fat is to use it as fuel. Yes, body fat is a food source.

Now, using some simple math and the standard that a pound of fat has roughly 3500 calories in it, if you had 25 pounds of fat you want to lose, which is what I have found to be a very common desire, you are looking at 87,500 calories as an energy source (3500 x 25).

That's a damn lot of energy. But here's the thing, if you are constantly fueling your body from an outside source, like most diets recommend with multiple small meals per day, you give your body no reason to tap into those 87 thousand plus calories.

Body fat is food. Allow the body to 'eat' it.

Another big point that I want to make is that you must think of traditional diets and fasting as two distinct and very different roads.

In a traditional setting, the so-called expert (fake fitness experts) would have you cut calories. Now, there are a few problems with this right off the bat.

First, they usually start you out blind, meaning they have no knowledge of what you are currently doing. And that can be a problem when we are talking about forming habits.

One of the main things that will put the brain into survival mode is when things are going too fast. I used to make this mistake all the time with clients.

I would calculate based on weight how much I thought they should be eating. A month or so would go by and some people wouldn't change at all. This meant either I gave them faulty advice or they weren't adhering to the plan.

It's much easier for the experts to pin the blame on the client/patient than to admit that what has been taught for decades is flat out wrong.

The Losing Proposition of Traditional Diets

The Calorie Game

Most 'diets' are centered on the flawed idea that we can lose weight by playing the calorie equation game. Cut calories and weight will drop. In the very short term, this is what can happen, although I've seen it fail even from the get go in myself and others.

The biggest part of our metabolism is what's known as our basal metabolic rate (BMR). This is basically the amount of energy our bodies will use while at rest, with no activity, to run all the systems of the body.

Think of your immune system, brain function, organ functioning, etc. There's a lot more to the body than just exercise and the muscular system.

A main Mind Map principle that you always have to remember is that everything your brain tells you and everything your body does internally is for survival first.

Point being, when you cut calories like most diets have you do, your body will down-regulate your BMR to match what you are putting in.

And, it has a pretty wide range of how far it can go; usually a 40% swing in either direction is normal in most people. This means that if you have a BMR of 2000 calories, you can cut up to 800 and essentially be eating around 1200 calories and not lose weight.

(To figure out your BMR, there are all types of fancy equations and machines like we have our Newell Strength facilities, but the simple way to do it that puts you pretty damn close in case you were curious is to simply take your bodyweight and multiply it by 10).

I've even seen it more drastic than that in some of our women clients.

Now, you go along and lose weight the first few weeks or months if you are lucky and are blessed with extreme motivation and willpower.

Then, all of the sudden, your weight loss stops. So, the Fake Fitness Expert that convinced you that this was the only way to do it (that is pretty much what 99% of doctors and fake fitness experts are going to tell you to do), which leads you to believe that you need to cut more.

You do that, but nothing happens and worse yet, your biofeedback signals such as appetite, hunger, performance, mindset and so on are telling you that you can't sustain it much longer.

And the reason you can't sustain it is a hormone called ghrelin. Ghrelin is your main hunger hormone.

The thing with traditional diets is that your metabolism comes down to match the input as already stated, meanwhile, your main hunger hormone, ghrelin, continues to rise the longer you are eating in a big deficit.

Now, listen, I don't care how much willpower you have, this hunger will overcome you.

When you go back to eating 'normal', you will have a bigger appetite than normal, such as I did in my Waffle House phase and your metabolism will be lowered. This is how people get themselves into the yo-yo weight gain and loss cycle.

Meanwhile, your body resets its set point to a higher number. We all have a set-point: The tight range that your body is capable of sustaining. For example, the lower end of your set-point might be 175 pounds.

If you force yourself through caloric deprivation like so many people do to try to get below that, your body will resist and reset. This is a protective mechanism for survival.

Remember, our bodies store fat primarily as a fuel source. When times get scarce, we need body fat to call upon as a readily available energy source.

The problem is, in today's day and age, we rarely have a scarcity of food, and we combine that with the faulty advice that keeps getting rammed down our throats and we wind up with the obesity epidemic that we now have.

I will continue to say it over and over again: we are not playing the calorie game! Fasting takes a completely different metabolic pathway than cutting calories.

If cutting calories worked, a person would only have to diet once and then they would be all set. And to all the fake fitness experts out there, if it worked, your client would have kept the weight off.

If they didn't, it didn't work.

Listen, in Mind Mapping, which I used to develop every aspect of this Panda Diet, combined with 2 decades of nutritional education and experience, the whole key is helping people transform.

• • • • •

'Dieting' and Willpower

I can remember back to when I was getting ready for my last bodybuilding show and sneaking downstairs late at night to have some almond butter.

It wasn't a part of my plan, but I couldn't help it.

I was deep into preparation and although I had started on the 16:8 fasting protocol, I was still basing my leaning out on severe calorie restriction.

So, here I am, an uber-disciplined dude, and I couldn't help it, the almond butter was calling to me.

I needed it, or so I thought.

Well, in actuality, what was happening was that I was burning through my willpower to such a large extent each day that I had no shot at resisting a late night snack because I was following the Fake Fitness Expert dogma is cut, cut, cut, but keep eating, just cut it way down.

The longer you try to use willpower to form a habit, the quicker you can be sure that you are going to fail.

You see, your brain will not form a habit around anything that is willpower based.

However, your brain will form a habit around something that it finds pleasurable to do.

The part of your brain, the prefrontal cortex (Mind Map), that largely uses willpower, is dependent on glucose.

Being that your brain accounts for about 25% of the body's total energy expenditure, and by the end of a day, when many other events and people have competed for your willpower, you can rest easy knowing that it doesn't have a fighting chance.

Now, on a regular plan of eating, willpower continues to decline, metabolism begins to slow and your main hunger hormones continue to climb.

Somehow adding those 3 things together doesn't seem to be a good idea.

Doing things with willpower means doing things that you don't want to do. Go back and remember that your brain will only form a habit around things of importance that it finds pleasurable to repeat on a consistent basis.

With a regular diet in which you continue to cut calories and never really eat any foods that you enjoy, you will accelerate your decline in willpower, which leads to a vicious cycle of you blaming yourself and thinking that nothing will ever work because you simply lack a strong will.

Any fake fitness expert out there that leads you to believe it is your fault—your inability to stick with a diet plan that they have prescribed—is a numbskull that doesn't understand fasting metabolism nor do they know a lick about Mind Map/brain science.

• • • • •

Charles Poliquin Embarrassing Me

Back in 2011 in Tempe, Arizona, I was pumped to be heading to a 4-day course to learn from the late, great, Charles Poliquin.

To give you a little background about Charles, he was the guru's guru. He had trained hundreds of professional athletes and had developed a system over the years known as BioSignature Modulation.

It was a very high level course, in which he used his findings from working with various doctors and functional medicine experts to put together a software tool where a practitioner such as me could take the skinfold measurement of 12 sites, enter them into the software and get very detailed readings.

The cool thing about it was that each site corresponded to a specific hormone in the body. It took him over 20,000 measurements and blood work profiles to develop this, so to say the man was a genius would be an understatement (he literally tested at genius level in 4 of the 8 human intelligences).

Anyhow, on day 2, when we got to the actual mechanics of how to measure a client, he asked me to come up, since I was sitting right in the front row.

You may think that since I had competed numerous times in bodybuilding in nothing more than essentially a speedo in front of thousands of people that this would have been no big deal.

The thing was, I followed a very disciplined lifestyle of training and nutrition, but I rarely looked like a bodybuilder unless it was right around show time and this classroom was full of fitness experts from around the country, all of whom looked to be in pretty darn good shape!

Of course, I had to take my shirt off, and then for the next 30 minutes, he proceeded to teach the class how to measure each site, while judging and taking shots at my body fat and shape the entire time. It was humiliating to say the least.

His advice was basically that I should stay away from any carb source, including most vegetables, for the better part of the next 6 months and then I could suck on a mint here and there.

This was crazy!!! Yet, I believe what he was saying because he was the guru. The thing was that I was already eating a pretty low carb, low calorie plan 6 days per week. I was training consistently and doing all the things that I had asked our clients to do.

I left Arizona feeling excited about what I had learned in the course and excited to put it to use on myself as well as the clients. I even stopped by a private laboratory on the way back home from my red eye flight to Philly that very next morning at 8 AM to get updated blood work.

Surely, I had now found the reasons that as Devon would say, 'I never looked like I should compared to my behaviors with eating and training'.

Make no mistake about it, I am not saying that a person has to be ripped and chiseled; fasting can certainly help you down that path if that is your desire, but that isn't for most of us for various reasons.

I, like you, wanted to feel more confident and to realize that my efforts were paying off.

Moving forward from Arizona I followed his prescription with diet to a T and also got on some exotic, magical supplements (more on my view on supplements later).

I was essentially doing what the rest of the industry was doing, watching calories, taking supplements and cutting out entire food groups. I left feeling that it was a matter of having more information (as if there weren't enough of this floating around). It was a matter of being more disciplined, using more willpower and adding in the magic combination of protein and those darn supplements.

Yes, that had to be the answer. It confirmed my understanding at the time that if a client wasn't getting their desired weight loss, it was clearly their lack of will and understanding.

Boy, what a 'numb-nutz' I was. I was a 'fake fitness expert', but to give myself credit, I was always learning and growing and doing the best I could at the time as a Coach.

The difference was that I always kept my 'empty my cup' philosophy, I reserved the right to change my mind as I tried and learned new things, unlike most of the fake fitness experts out there.

• • • • •

Emptying Your Cup

How did I wind up being a fitness renegade? Well, my parents would tell you that I was always stubborn, persistent, and know it all.

When you mix these 3 things together, you create someone that has an insatiable thirst for knowledge. Here's the thing with knowledge: if your proverbial cup is always full and you are married to the ways you have always done things, then you will have no room to put any new information in.

I have tried damn near everything in fitness and I realized that in the end, it all came down to the simple, not the complex.

I used to believe in high protein, eating multiple times per day, keeping carbs low and on and on.

If I didn't live by the principle of the empty cup, then this book wouldn't be here right now.

Surprisingly, Charles Poliquin passed away about a year ago at the age of 57.

• • • • •

My Record Breaking Day at Waffle House

It was August of 2014. In fact, I remember the exact date because it happened to be my birthday, August the 10th.

Just 6 weeks prior, I had competed in two different bodybuilding shows a week apart.

Now, although I had just begun my fasting quest, my approach to getting into contest shape was extreme and based around cutting calories.

From creating 'metabolic damage' through my prior years of competing, I would have to eat at 1500-1700 calories per day with super hard workouts to drop my body fat levels to the level I needed to be contest ready.

Now, I understand that you are most likely not interested in bodybuilding and that's fine.

But I did learn from the extremes.

I'll circle back to the physiological benefits of fasting later and what I first noticed while starting short form fasting during this time period; but for now, back to August the 10th.

I had been dieting for close to 4.5 months on a big deficit of food. What made it somewhat tolerable was the fact that I knew how the human body's metabolism worked and I knew that to completely not shut down I would have to spike my calories once per week or so.

This was my 'cheat day' and when I tell you they were insane, that doesn't come close to describing them.

Yes, I had decided to continue my extreme 'cycle diet' for the remainder of that summer of 2014 because I was already in peak shape so I thought I might as well continue with it for the remainder of the summer until we went on our family vacation to the OBX in North Carolina.

For my cheat day, we left the house for the long day's drive down to Carolina at 6 AM.

While still in town we stopped by the local D and D and picked up a dozen double chocolate donuts. I finished them while driving before we got to the next town.

Then, while riding through Delaware and Maryland, I ate a quart of homemade rice pudding that Devon had made for me and a large bag of Butterfingers.

I know, at this point you are probably thinking this was crazy and it was, but stay with me.

We get down to Virginia Beach and had already scouted out a Waffle House, one of my favorite treats since we don't have them in Jersey.

By this time, it was around 11 AM.

The place looked to be packed. My only instruction to Devon was, 'Please don't tell them it's my birthday. You know I don't like to be the center of attention.'

I should have figured that was not the reason people would be paying attention to me on this particular visit.

We sat down, got some coffees and placed our order. Devon did her thing and then I ordered: 'I'll start with some eggs and 3 peanut butter waffles please.'

The waitress said, 'I'm sorry, I thought you said 3 waffles.' To which I confirmed that indeed I had.

She started laughing and telling the other waitresses. The commotion had started.

Meanwhile, there was a dad and son sitting next to me that saw I was wearing one of my old Rutgers Strength and Conditioning shirts from my time there in the early 2000's.

The dad was nice enough and started asking me nutrition and training questions for his son, an aspiring varsity football player.

I am answering their questions as we sat at the 'bar', again the place was packed. When my food came out, the dad started laughing out loud. I tried to briefly explain to him what I am going to explain to you in a minute.

But my main focus was on eating those waffles!

Needless to say, I downed the waffles and eggs as easy as 1-2-3.

So, that early commotion had now turned into essentially a standing ovation. Hey, I couldn't let the people down and I was still hungry (remember this, that is the point I am going to illustrate). To which I ordered 2 more giant, peanut butter waffles.

I thought the waitress would faint!

She starts telling me that she had never seen anyone eat more than 2 in a sitting. She couldn't fathom an appetite like mine existed, especially for the kind of shape that I was in; essentially in near bodybuilding shape because of the contests a few weeks prior.

By this point, there was an electric buzz in my corner of the restaurant. People had started to gather around.

The waffles came out and I went to work. Now, keep in mind how much I had already eaten that morning.

As I was nearly finished with the 5th giant waffle, the manager came out. He offered to buy our meal if I ordered 2 more and was able to finish them.

I politely declined because I realized that while I could have done it, the rest of my drive would have been spent in a near food coma.

I did get a hat out of it and a picture with the staff.

I felt like John Candy eating the old 96er in the 80's hit, The Great Outdoors.

I won't bore you with how much I ate that night for my birthday celebration because it's the same sort of deal.

Ok, so the point of this, and yes, there was a point (Mind Map principle: the brain learns and remembers best through stories) was that I had created what one of my former mentors calls a 'supercompensation' mode.

Normally, I have a big appetite but can eat nowhere near as much as I did on that particular birthday.

So how did I do it? Well, you no doubt have experienced a similar thing just to a less extreme degree. I did it by cutting calories for an extended amount of time while working out too much.

• • • • •

The Consequences of Bad Dieting

I am not going to make this point overly long, because I just want to drive home a couple of key points.

When you 'diet' incorrectly:

- Your hunger will continue to rise over time with a corresponding ability to eat more
- You will burn through willpower
- You will train your body to reset its body weight set point higher and higher to fight against the next time you play the calorie game
- You will feel guilty because of your lack of adherence
- You will lose weight, then proceed to gain it all back and then some (refer to set point above)
- You will cut out entire food groups, which inevitably will make you crave them and want them more → you will eat them, gain weight and claim that you are 'carb sensitive' or something of the like

Yup, that about sums it up.

Retraining Your Mind

Mind Mapping Primer

One main thing that makes the Panda 'Diet' so great is that I have infused it with Mind Mapping principles. In short, Mind Mapping is the actual neuroscience of habit formation and something that very few people in the world are experts at. Luckily for you, I am one of the few Mind Map experts in the world.

I do plan on writing an entire book on Mind Map at some point soon, but for our intents and purposes, I want to give you an overview of it.

One of the main Mind Map principles is to gain clarity. If we don't have clarity, the mind will not allow us to move forward and act.

Information is rarely, if ever the problem. In this case, if a lack of information regarding what to eat was the problem, a quick Google search would solve that for you.

So, if information isn't the problem, then why can't people reach and sustain their ultimate goals?

It is because of something known as the triune brain theory. Basically, you and I have 3 layers of the brain: the reptilian brain, the mammalian brain and the human brain (frontal cortex).

It is within the human brain that we set goals, have logical, linear thought and the desire to reach self-actualization.
The problem is that there are often threats and stresses to the mammal brain that keep pulling us out of our human mind, which means we cannot maintain focus long enough on a new habit to move it deeper into our brain where it becomes permanent.

Problems in your environments or your relationships need to be addressed and cleared up first otherwise, the old patterns will continue to surface, leaving no room for your new habits.

There are 3 things that put the brain into threat: when things are going too fast, when things are going too slowly and when there is unclear intent.

- Too fast
- Too slow
- Lack of clarity

Think about how this applies to most diets. People go from no structure to having way too much structure, in a micro-obsessed way. They are told to eat 5-6x times per day, they have to measure their food and they have to figure out how to cook all of this stuff.

In this particular case, that was too fast for most people and way too unclear.

Now, think about if you've been trying to lose those 15-30 pounds for what seems like years. You lose it, you gain it, you lose it, you gain it, and so on. This will make us go into 'threat mode' because it's simply too slow.

The human brain isn't getting to realize it's self-actualizing goal of achieving that weight loss.

Mind Map follows 12 steps:

1. Provides safety
2. Safety allows for exploration
3. Exploration allows for clarity
4. Clarity allows for understanding
5. Understanding leads to belief
6. Belief leads to trust
7. Trust leads to action
8. Action leads to change
9. Change leads to habit
10. Habit leads to transformation
11. Transformation leads to growth
12. Growth leads us back into new threats

It is my hope that by being 'your Coach', you start down the path with safety which eventually leads us to your transformation.

You may be wondering why growth would lead to new threats.

It's simple. The human mind thrives on growth, it makes it happy. Growth leads us to explore new things that we have no mastery of which will lead us to new threats and we will begin the process all over again.

A change is temporary.

A transformation is permanent.

• • • • •

The Pendulum Effect

Anytime in life that we force the body to do something, we experience what I call the pendulum effect.

I first learned this once again with my competition days. In bodybuilding, its common practice to do extreme and drastic things right before contest day in the hopes of looking just a little bit better.

Things like completely cutting out water, completely cutting out salts, completely cutting out carbs and the list goes on.

And I have seen this in so many instances throughout the years with regular trainees and clients. They decide to swear off carbs, go 'keto', cut calories in half and so on.

I always cringe when I hear this because as I learned with bodybuilding, anytime you force the body to do something extreme, the pendulum will swing all the way towards that side, but what people fail to realize is that the pendulum will swing back, equally and oppositely just as extreme.

The only difference being you cannot predict when that will happen; we only know that it will happen.

How many times have you or someone you knew swore that you were sensitive to carbs? Listen; if you had the genetics that made you sensitive to carbs, you wouldn't be here.

And that's because your ancestors would not have survived. Everything the body does is for survival first and foremost.

Carbs were and always will be the most easily and readily food source.

The reason people swear that they are carb sensitive is because they have bought into all the nonsense about carbs being evil, which lead them to cutting out carbs or drastically reducing them and then when they can no longer take it, they reintroduce them or 'binge' and they blow up like a swollen tick engorged with blood.

This is not carb sensitivity; it's the pendulum effect and a little basic physiology.

Without getting too technical and to be honest, I don't even know the names of some of the specific enzymes (nor does it matter), enzyme activity for storage of things like glycogen goes up when you cut carbs for a period of time.

This is the reason some runners used to and some still do, practice carb loading, which has to be preceded by a period of carb depletion (pendulum effect again!).

If you deplete, your ability to store more temporarily goes up.

And when it comes to the recreational dieter, such as yourself, looking to lose weight, you might get all giddy about early results when you go low carb or try the dreaded KETO plan. But once you realize that every gram of carbohydrate combines with 3 grams of water in the body to form glycogen, then you realize that if you cut carbs, you cut water weight, which is pointless in most instances.

Remember my experience at the Waffle House. That was simply a matter of extreme depletion and manipulating hormones to have that monstrous of an eating capacity.

The main points I want you to internalize with the pendulum effect are these:

- When you do anything that involves extreme willpower you can be sure that you are activating the supercompensation system of the pendulum effect. And if it involves extreme willpower, you can be sure that it violates the basic premise of any good plan, which I wrote about earlier in that it must be functional and sustainable (forever!).

- Your brain will not form a habit around anything that it doesn't find pleasurable. That would go against the very concept of comfort and survival that the brain craves.

- The pendulum will swing back just as hard and just as far as you decided to push it with your New Year's Resolution or faulty plan that your local fake fitness expert put you on

If you internalize this, you know more about nutrition than most so called experts. It is fundamental physiology.

Don't let anyone come in and confuse you with fancy terms of why their theoretical concepts work because of science. We here with the Panda Diet system are interested in lasting results and true transformations!

The History of Breakfast

The Misconception of Breakfast

If there is one main 'enemy' of fasting, it is the concept of the traditional breakfast.

We've all been told that it is the most important meal of the day.

We've been told that breakfast gets the metabolism going.

And it's all a big bunch of BS!

Charles Poliquin first taught me about the 'fisching effect' which states that insulin and cortisol have an opposing relationship in many ways.

What this effect states is that lets say cortisol is high and you consume food that is going to cause an increase in insulin, then an hour or two later, cortisol levels will drop.

So, what's the problem with that? It is a good question, and one that I will address before I get into the history of breakfast.

If you look at the circadian rhythm of the human body, it has natural cycles all across the board.

For our intents and purposes, let's focus on cortisol. Cortisol should begin to rise an hour or so before wake and hit its peak between 6-8 am. Now, in some people, this is reversed and they have high cortisol levels at night, which is another issue altogether and is not normal.

However, to stay on track, cortisol is the main alertness hormone that we have.

From Mind Map, I learned that the most stressful physiological time of the day for the human body is upon waking.

Think about it, you are going from a sleep state to a conscious state. Now consider that, yes, we wake up in nice comfortable beds nowadays, within the shelter of our homes.

But it wasn't always this way. If you went back thousands of years and or even longer, upon waking, you would have to gather your bearings, account for your family, locate any threats and then get ready to hunt and gather so that you could survive.

We wanted cortisol to be high during this time of day.

Going back to the fisching effect: if we eat a typical breakfast, we will get an insulin response, which will cause cortisol to come back down a while later. That is not a good thing, if we want the weight loss effects and health effects of fasting.

If we allow cortisol to continue to rise, growth hormone will rise along with it. The longer we get into a fast, the more growth hormone output we get. Both cortisol and growth hormone are profound in their ability to help us 'burn' stored body fat. Both are also excellent for brain sharpness and mental clarity.

When you examine the myth of breakfast from this standpoint, it becomes blazingly obvious that it doesn't go hand in hand with the hormones of our body.

Most people that eat the typical North American diet will complain of hunger and lethargy shortly after eating what they thought was a health breakfast is because of the insulin response and insulin decline that will follow sometime after.

Here's an interesting thing about insulin and cortisol. Cortisol can either be profound in its ability to help us use stored body fat or it can be very fat-storing friendly.

How can it be both? Well, in the presence of high insulin levels, cortisol will lead to more inflammation and a greatly increased ability to store fat.

But, you say, 'how can they both be high at the same time?' When we aren't dealing with our stress correctly and those stress signals an excessive release of the fight or flight hormones known as cortisol and adrenaline, then we will have a constant flow of those hormones.

Combine this with the fact most people eat multiple times per day and when they are stressed, they eat low-quality foods loaded with saturated fat and sugar and the problem just continues to get worse, day after day.

This explains why one person can be extremely stressed and actually lose weight, while another person can be extremely stressed and gain a ton of weight. The former responds to cortisol with a suppressed appetite the latter responds to cortisol with an increase in appetite.

Now that you know more about the cortisol and insulin hormones than most doctors, let me go into a brief history of breakfast.

Remember, this is all about Mind Mapping, and you connecting the dots. If you don't connect the dots yourself, then you'll never be able to form a long term habit around the practice of fasting or any other habit for that matter. Clarity leads to trusting the process, trusting the process leads to further action.

• • • • •

A Brief History of Breakfast

In Europe, breakfast was only for those that worked so early that they had to get the fuel into their body for the long day ahead; otherwise they would have to wait until dinner (which wouldn't have been a bad thing in my humble but accurate opinion). In addition, breakfast was recommended to the elderly and the sickly, in order to help them keep weight on and get in vital micronutrients.

I am guessing that since the elderly and sickly have a reduced appetite, the thought was that they had to have smaller feedings spread throughout the day in order to meet a minimum standard. I don't agree with it but I do understand the line of thought.

Historian Ian Mortimer also believed that in 16th century Europe, breakfast was a side effect of employment, in which the worker lost control of their time because of having to work long, uninterrupted hours (remember, this was long before unions existed). Eating beforehand or waiting until the night to eat were their only options.

So, as we can see, it was a thing of believed necessity at first, but how did it then become something of an emotional attachment and when did this happen?

In the 19th century, Dr. John Harvey Kellogg (the name should look familiar), developed a granola and cornflakes cereal as part of a puritan diet designed to suppress sexual desire and lead America away from sin and masturbation.

This sounds absurd but it's true.

One of Kellogg's top workers, Charles M. Post, left and founded Grape Nuts and then Post Cereal and the cereal race was on.

This meant a few things. The mass marketing machine would eventually take hold and if you know anything about marketing, you'll know that it is based in emotion, not logic. People buy into the emotional need for things, they don't buy on logic.

If you hear that message long enough then you wind up where we are: believing that breakfast is the most important meal of the day. Now, add to that the fact that cereal was very convenient because it takes zero prep time and it wasn't long before other foods that were super easy to prepare began to take hold such as bagels, donuts and muffins.

Around the time of WWI, Orange Juice began to be pushed because of the Spanish Flu making people more aware of vitamins. The only problem is that orange juice is pretty much like drinking straight, simple sugar. You lose the fiber and for most, it's artificial coloring and flavoring. Yet, people have bought into the idea that orange juice should be a staple in the morning.

In the 1920's, public relations expert, Edward Bernay, was trying to help the company he worked for, Beech & Nut, sell bacon. He figured the easiest way to do this was to link it up with another staple: eggs. Bernay convinced 5,000 doctors to sign a letter recommending bacon and eggs as a healthy breakfast.

I wanted to go through all of this so you have an understanding of the history of what you've been led to believe. Without clarity, there can be no trust in the process. Without trust, there can be no true transformation.

Hopefully that sheds some light on where breakfast came from and how it came to be known as the most important meal of the day.

• • • • •

The Idea of Eating Every Few Hours

This goes hand in hand with breakfast.

Do you know who funds the studies that have said we must eat every few hours? Food and supplement companies, that's who!

And the theory has been repeated by buffed up bodybuilders masquerading as trainers for no other reason than the fact they were told that's what they should do, so they repeated it.

People mistake the hunger feeling they get with eating frequently as a revved up metabolism. That's not at all what that is. It's simply the entrainment pattern driving more frequent hunger signals.

Listen; there is simply no money for these companies to make off people that live a fasting focused lifestyle.

Follow the dollar and you can guess who came up with damn near all of the traditional nutrition dogma.

Fasting and Fear

To understand why so many people are fearful of fasting, we need to understand one of the main philosophies of Mind Map.

And that is this: a lack of clarity will cause us to go into a survival response.

The brain thrives on patterns (prediction + response).

With fasting, we have been told all these big, scary lies that it will shut our body down, we will enter starvation mode, we will get shaky because of low blood sugar and we will suffer from low energy.

Understandably, people have a lot of fear around fasting.

Fear is based on future-based thought. The future is a figment of our imagination (think about that for a second, it's mind-blowing). The future literally does not exist besides our imagination of what might happen at a later date and time.

When it comes to fasting, we think about all the things that could possibly go wrong, all the things we have been told by the fake fitness experts.

It's a fear of the unknown. This is a big part of why I have many clients start out with a 48-hour fast right out of the gait; it builds confidence.

And a big part of the fear is that we can't imagine going without food for an extended period of time because of the emotional comfort food provides us.

We've been told that we need food for energy and that we shouldn't let our blood sugar drop.

Believe me, there is no one that enjoys food as much as I, but that is when we have to keep in mind the context of what food is and the 'food is a drug' aspect mentality.

As with anything I write about, I believe that you cannot take advice from a so-called 'expert' that hasn't done the very act themselves.

They will want to tell you how bad it is for you without having tried it themselves which is one of the big signs of being a fake fitness expert.

Many people have been led to believe that they will go 'hypoglycemic' (low blood sugar), which is rarely a concern. I will admit that diabetics on certain medications need to keep an eye on this when they first begin on their fasting journey but for a normal person looking to drop weight, low blood sugar isn't a real threat.

Just as when blood sugar is too high, your body releases insulin to handle it and shuttle it for storage, your body has another hormone called glucagon that will ramp up when your body senses blood sugar dropping.

Yes, glucagon will not let you dip below a certain level and the cool thing is that glucagon needs to be present for fat loss to happen!

Listen clearly, DO NOT take advice on fasting from a fitness 'expert' that has never tried fasting for an extended period of time, they simply cannot speak on it from a place of wisdom and truth.

Fasting and Hunger

During that same summer that I became a legend at the Waffle House, we went away for the night to a place up in northern New Jersey.

And yes, of course, I had it planned so it fell on one of my 'cheat days'. Well, actually, at that point I had it scheduled so that I had a 'cheat night', usually on a Thursday and then a full day on Sundays.

In case you didn't catch on with the Waffle House story, my normally huge capacity to eat was heightened greatly because of how I had 'trained' my body by how I had been eating that summer.

This meant that to be able to bear the hunger on the other days, I had to really make sure I took in a ton of food on my 1 and a half cheat days each week.

Ok, so we go out to this bar/restaurant and I proceed to order 3 appetizers, two burger platters, 3 extra sides and a milkshake. The waitress assumed I had ordered for both Devon and I, to which we had to inform her that nope, that was just for me.

She was dumbfounded and she kept looking around the corner to see if I was actually eating all the food. She couldn't fathom an appetite such as she was seeing and I laughed, not even trying to explain my current metabolic state to her at the time.

(We went out for dessert afterwards. ☺)

Well, the point here is that by drastically reducing calories on my 'diet', my hunger continually climbed but more importantly for this point I want to make is that my eating capacity rose right alongside my hunger.

I can tell you that as I sit here and write this that there is no way I could eat that much food in one sitting anymore.

Because, when you fast correctly, for longer periods of time, like you would here with this Panda Diet, your hunger does not go up.

It actually decreases over time. And being that hunger actually declines, appetite doesn't rise nearly as much you would think it would.

Hunger as most people know it is merely a psychological trigger.

In fact, I am writing this entry on a Monday night, which means I am in the middle of my weekly 48-hour fast and just writing about those great eating memories is triggering a hunger response. But I know it'll pass in a minute or two.

With fasting, it is super important to keep in mind that our body fat is 'food'. When you feel hunger, you must reframe it as 'this is what weight loss/fat loss' feels like and know that it will pass very quickly.

People are very quick to mistake this 'Pavlov's dogs' effect with actual, true, hunger. Remember, as I spoke about before, the entrainment patterns. Over the years, you've trained your body when to expect food and you will be damn sure to get hungry at those times, especially when you first start out.

Most people get 'hangry' if they, god-forbid, go more than a few hours without eating. We need to stop this insanity!!!

It takes the body roughly 6-hours after a meal to enter a fasted state. And it's important to know that according to the Panda Diet philosophy, there is a duality to eating: we are either in a fed or fasted state, either in an anabolic or catabolic state, there is no in-between.

So, how is it logically possible that we are in true hunger a few hours after eating if we are still in a 'fed state'?

Well, it's not logically possible, but it is emotionally possible.

We are constantly triggered by environmental cues, social cues and marketing to desire and crave food. Do not confuse this with actual, real hunger.

The U.S. food industry spends $10 billion per year on advertising and it works! In a recent *New England Journal of Medicine* paper I was reading, the doctors concurred about all the health benefits of fasting and are now pumping out research left and right to back it up.

But they finish with: 'We will be hard pressed to ever make this mainstream because of the mass marketing we face that flies in the face of this research.'

Remember, food is a drug and according to another article in *Scientific Mind*, drug addiction and binge eating are very similar in 'neurobiological terms'. Your brain reacts to food (not only sugar) the same way a cocaine addict's brain would react to cocaine.

Now, there are a couple of key points here. Of particular importance is the word *reacts*, not *responds*. The deeper part of your brain—the part where habit is held; the animal brains—*reacts*, it does not *respond*.

This means that of course, we know something to be true logically, but logic and emotion do not mix. I am sure you have every intention of not snacking on chips and cookies late at night, but when that time rolls around, you have no shot.

This ties in very nicely to the idea that regular diets are set up to fail, because they are based in willpower and anything that is willpower based is doomed to fail. First, because willpower is doing something you don't really want to do. Second, the prefrontal cortex region of our brain—where willpower is held—is extremely energy hungry.

This means that by the end of the day, after dealing with work and any other family responsibilities, your willpower is gone, it's spent for the day. Willpower is a very finite resource.

When willpower is spent for the day, you can kiss your good intentions goodbye.

Let's revisit this idea of hunger and fasting. It does take a degree of self-awareness and self-mastery, both of which can be learned because they are both skills.

All skills can be learned.

But realize that when you decide to pop open that cookie jar, it is the drug aspect of the food that is causing you to do that, not actual hunger.

From the time you were a little baby, when you cried, your mom fed you milk, either from the bottle or her boob, but the point remains, a dose of food is wired to be calming to us from the time we are newborns.

If you combine the drug aspect of food along with the mass marketing machine that the food and supplement industry is, you realize that you are in for quite the battle.

I will tell you that the way I have designed the Panda Diet gives you a great chance to be successful because I have incorporated so many Mind Map principles into it.

Fasting and Gut Health

Giving Your Gut a Break

Back in the very same classroom that Charles Poliquin roasted me in front of everyone, I actually did take copious notes and learned a thing or three.

One of the main things that stuck with me is that gut health and digestion are paramount to health.

In fact, I would argue that for young to middle aged men, if they have regular, consistent bowel movements and can get an erection, then their health is pretty damn good. For women, I would say that swap out erection with a regular menstrual cycle and they are spot on then too.

Anyhow, our main digestive enzyme, hydrochloric acid, HCL, is depleted by stress.

Charles gave us a pack of HCL pills and instructed us how to run the 'test' over the next day or so. At every meal, you would take one pill in the middle of the meal, and if you didn't feel anything, then would up it by one pill at the next meal and so on.

I believe at the time, you could work up to five-7 pills and as you 'turned' on your HCL over time, you would get a burning sensation which would signal you to decrease the dose by one pill.

Well, I never got that burning sensation, even after moving to the stronger pills.

Until that is, I began fasting. Within the first month, I started realizing that I was getting a burning after eating, totally foreign to me.

It clicked! Fasting was allowing my gut a break! I was allowing the enzymes to replenish!

One of the main things with fasting is that it reduces inflammation globally throughout the body, but no place more important than in your stomach.

With all that said, fasting should improve digestion and help with issues such as 'acid reflux'.

• • • • •

Jabba

In 1989, I met one of my very best friends. It's a hell of a thing when I am 38 years old and I have a friend that I met over 30 years ago.

Anyway, we call him Jabba.

About a year ago, Jabba approached me because he was getting worried about his health. Now, if you knew Jabba, you would know that this is something he would only do if he were truly worried.

So, I got him going on a fasting program straight away.

And he proceeded to lose 30 or so pounds in relatively short order.

But that is not the most impressive part.

For as long as I can remember, Jabba has had GI inflammation, indigestion, ulcers and bloating.

The doctor has had him on Nexium for years and to no avail. Now, once again, I am not a doctor but I have made my life's work of studying the human body.

As best as I can understand indigestion and heartburn, it is not a problem of too much acid, rather, it is a problem of too little acid (HCL, which I spoke about earlier).

So, you may be asking, why do you get reflux then? Simple, because your HCL is low, your ability to break down and digest your food fully is lowered. The food sits there longer than it should, ferments and wants to escape upwards.

The sphincter of the esophagus opens and some of that partially digested foodstuff which does have some stomach acid mixed with it, comes back up, and burns.

Prescribing you Nexium or the like only makes problems worse.

Back to Jabba. In addition to dropping the weight, he recently had his one year check up with his GI doctor. The doctor performed an endoscopy and reported that there was no longer any inflammation. Let me repeat that, NONE, NADA, ZERO!

To which the doctor was very curious about and then he told Jabba that he thought they would be able to cut back his medication to half the dose, to which Jabba replied that he had already been off of it for a couple of months.

How is this possible?

I'll get to that in a second, but realize that for gut health, fasting and drinking the juice, your salt water mix will work wonders on healing the inflammation in your gut.

Inflammation is a sign that something is wrong. It is also the start of every disease. With inflammation, you can be sure to find its cousin, insulin resistance, lurking nearby.

There are a few different paths to this. First, most people are overly stressed as I mentioned earlier. They spend most of their time being in a survival mode of fight, flight or freeze. This alone, will cause inflammation.

Now add to that that most people eat while in this state, which leads to further insulin resistance, which leads to more inflammation.

And in the case of your gut, when you are constantly eating and not giving it a break, it will lead to inflammation.

What if you were to go in and train your back muscles or arms every couple of hours, much like people do to their gut when they are eating? You wouldn't ever recover because you would have chronic inflammation. The same logic applies to your gut.

As I mentioned earlier, when I first began fasting with a 16:8 protocol, one of the first things I noticed was that I was able to stop taking my HCL pills. There was a specific protocol in which to take them, but once you started to feel a mild burn, you knew you no longer needed them because your own system was 'back online'.

Remember, one of the best and quickest ways to reduce overall inflammation in the body is to fast.

Here are two empirical accounts, one from my good friend and proofreader of this book, Drew:

'My seasonal allergies disappeared this year and the only thing different in my life is that I switched to OMAD.'

And another from a client of ours at Newell Strength named Linda: 'I've had chronic sinusitis for as long as I can remember. I can tell you that between supplementing with the juice and following the Panda fasting, it's damn near gone. A HUGE improvement! I have always had a whistling or whisping in my chest. I've always felt and heard it after laughing. It's gone! And the arthritis pain and stinging in my finger joints is gone!'

I know two random examples don't hold up to scientific scrutiny, but these are the types of stories I've heard from literally hundreds of clients over the past 5 years. I'll let you be the judge.

You are only as healthy as your gut health and it ties in nicely with your brain health. Your gut is called the second brain for a reason. Most of your serotonin is produced there along with many other neuro-hormones.

But, they can't do their jobs correctly if their house is constantly on fire.

Now you know where the term, 'gut-feeling', came from.

Fasting and Malnourishment

Do I Need to Meet a Calorie Minimum?

My sister in-law recently replied to a post I put up in our 'Fasting for Fitness' FB group in which I asked, 'What is your number 1 question as it relates to fasting right now?'

Taryn, my sister in law, had a common question, 'How can I make sure I am getting all my calories in if I am only eating one time per day?

Well, here's the thing: that line of thought comes from the traditional spew of calories in and calories out.

You and I, as I have shown, have pretty much for our intents and purposes, an unlimited number of calories stored on our body in the form of body fat.

Trying to fit in calories sake (unless weight gain is the goal) is senseless. Your body will take form its own stores to make up whatever energy supply you need during your fasting state.

It takes us about 6 hours or so after a meal to enter a fasted state, by the way.

And this ties in nicely to one of the main principles I learned from one of my Coaches long ago about bio-feedback. This is the awareness to listen to what your body is telling you. At first, for most, it takes a master Coach to be able to help with this with the correct questions and knowing what to look for.

Biofeedback is about the lead indicators, rather than eating to a number. Eating to a number is taking the outside in approach. Eating from the inside out is taking a mindful approach.

I just had a client reach out earlier this morning about his Panda Diet plan, which I monitor remotely since he lives a few hours away, (down 25 pounds and feeling great I'd like to add) and he wanted to know about how much to eat.

"Kyle, some nights, I get full very quickly. Some nights, I am ravenous."

Well, this is where you need to listen to those signals. To ignore them, like the FFEs would have you do it, is ludicrous.

Over time, with fasting, you will see this ability greatly improve.

So, for biofeedback, you have to look at such things as:

- appetite
- hunger
- energy in the gym and outside the gym
- performance in all phases of life
- sleep
- bathroom habits
- attitude

- mindset and mental clarity

When you are following the Panda Diet, you don't need to hit a certain macro count or hit a minimum or maximum amount of calories. That is something that can be addressed if needed but I have found to be a very distant secondary component.

It's more about when you eat rather than what you are eating.

I can hear the FFEs getting their pitchforks ready to come and get me right now. ☺

Which brings me to another funny story....

• • • • •

Don't I Have to Worry About Malnourishment?

A few weeks ago, in our Fasting FB group, a personal trainer started lecturing people about being malnourished and how you can't and shouldn't fast.

He was implying that trying to live a lifestyle where you eat once per day would lead to undereating of nutrients and therefore malnourishment.

And by the way, fake fitness experts love to use words like 'malnourished' and usually they have no real understanding of what the concept means.

Well, I asked, 'When's the last time that you saw anyone in the United States that was malnourished?'

Now, as an aside, I was trapping him in his own logic, which he didn't see coming.

He replied with, 'So you are telling me that overweight people can't be malnourished?'

Got him!

I went on to explain that first off, he was specifically referring to people being malnourished because of undereating.

Obese and overweight people aren't overweight from undereating; they are malnourished because they eat too frequently.

As you can see, he tried to flip his argument but I still wasn't done. I went on to explain that yes of course, many overweight people are malnourished but it's from something known as 'internal starvation'.

Internal starvation happens when we become more insulin resistant, specifically from a lack of sodium. Sodium is so critical to the functioning of each and every cell of our body that when we lack, we increase insulin to help us retain that which we do have.

In this instance, the insulin is also trapping not only sodium in the cell, but other vital nutrients, that we actually have in plentiful amounts in our body fat stores, but yet, we cannot access because of this internal starvation.

And that my friend, is how overweight and obese people become malnourished. Because remember, they are already creating insulin resistance through how often and what they eat, now you go and add a lack of sodium and *violà*!

• • • • •

Throwing a Ball

Just the other day, I was super excited because it was the first time that Braxton had shown an interest in basketball. We were up in the cul-de-sac and he was about to set up his army guys on the curb when he saw me dribbling a ball, while pushing Emma in her stroller.

He came over and said he wanted to try and next thing you know, I brought up the 6-foot, old school, glass backboard hoop from Brookstone that my brothers and I had as a kid.

We began to play and he even said, 'Dad, I'm Michigan State and you're the white team.' Very observant that little dude is, he knows that I love watching Michigan State hoops.

Anyhow, he proceeded to make a few baskets which made us both jump for joy!

Now, I want you to think back to the first time you threw a ball. Or if sports weren't your thing, think back to the first time you rode a bike and transpose that experience with throwing a ball.

If I were to instruct you to contract this medial muscle while making sure this tendon in your foot did that while making sure you turned your head that way and so on, you would think I was crazy. Weird, yes. But not crazy.

That's not how the body works. It simply moves and the inner intelligence of the body takes over.

The reason I thought about this is because I was recently asked about how your body knows how much of each nutrient it needs and how it knows when to store calories as fat and when to use calories for fuel.

And then there was the question of how much it could store in one meal.

Listen, your body has a beautiful inner working that knows how to do this automatically.

Most fake fitness experts and doctors teach nutrition in a reductionist way, much like me trying to instruct Braxton how to throw a ball by telling what muscle should be contracting during each phase.

Sorry, that doesn't work.

Take in the food and let the body do the work. Now, if you are feeding multiple times per day, then you are throwing everything off. As I have said before, insulin will signal to your body to store, store, store.

It is going to be damn near impossible to become malnourished eating in this fashion, just as it would be if you were eating your 3 square meals per day. And being malnourished is a boogeyman.

Think about this reality math for a second: have you ever seen a malnourished person in the civilized western world?

And, if it were to happen, it wouldn't happen overnight, just like you don't get fat or put on muscle overnight.

This feeds right into the fear-mongering that the FFE continues to propagate that if you don't eat every few hours your muscles will melt away, you'll become deficient in nutrients and on and on. Your cells have more nutrients stored in them than you can imagine but many times they stay locked away because we aren't accessing those storage units because of.

• • • • •

Shakes Are For Fakes

Back in my sophomore year and junior years of high school, my brothers and I convinced my mom to buy us 'mass gainer shakes'.

I used to have one of these once or twice per day, after a meal. They were a couple of thousand calories each and the taste was damn near unbearable.

I used to have to plug my nose for every sip; otherwise I couldn't get it down.

As you can see my self-experimentation has been going on for quite some time.

Now, if I knew then what I knew now, I wouldn't have been doing it. I was still under the assumption that I need protein and lots of it, which of course, I was led to believe, would be impossible just through eating whole foods.

Actually, while I am thinking of it, I got ready for two bodybuilding shows in 2007 without doing one single protein shake and as fate would have it, that was the best year of my competitive career.

I didn't lose a damn bit of muscle and I didn't because I trained damn hard.

Anyhow, here's the thing with fasting and shakes: we want to eat less often, not more and we don't need to supplement protein nor should we be eating on the run.

I always chuckle now when people ask me about shakes because I've been there and I totally get how they've been duped into buying into the whole concept.

Fasting by its very nature demands that we have less frequent feedings. So, if you are having less frequent feedings, why would you want to fill one of those gaps with a shake 'on the run'?

Look at it this way, a shake either means you are trying to get 'extra' in or you simply don't have time to sit and actually eat a meal, both of which are big no-no's in my book.

• • • • •

Go Primal

In March of 2020, the country and the world went on a worldwide quarantine because of the Coronavirus. I have many thoughts about that which you can probably surmise just by philosophy mentioned above. But I won't get into that because I don't want the point I want to make to get lost in my theory of these strange times.

One of the things that has happened is the mass hysteria is causing people to hoard grocery stores.

Which led me to think, 'What would people do if they couldn't get food at the grocery stores anymore'?

Fasting activates many primal traits, including hormesis. Hormesis is when we subject ourselves to constant mild stressors in order to grow physiologically more resistant and to become mentally tougher.

Modern society has made people too soft in my humble but accurate opinion. While we can't do many of the primal things our ancestors did, nor is there a need to do much of that stuff, we can still activate a little bit of it through the art of fasting.

Fasting and Weight Loss

I am sure you are wondering how fasting is different in terms of weight loss than cutting calories.

Let me explain that to you through an analogy.

Picture that you have a fridge in your kitchen that represents your body's energy stores (remember, the main purpose of glycogen and body fat is that it is to be used as a fuel source).

Now, that fridge is fully stocked to the gills.

You also have a few freezers down in the basement. They represent the excess weight that you would like to lose.

The problem is that you can't begin to tap into those freezers until you empty out the fridge upstairs.

The traditional approach to weight loss spewed out by the masses is that weight loss is simultaneous; meaning that if you take in fewer calories and burn more, then math says you will lose weight (even if your fridge is still semi-full upstairs!!!).

Well, the whole point of this book and my Panda Diet philosophy is that this approach is completely wrong!!!

Weight loss is sequential, meaning that your upstairs fridge has to be damn near empty and rarely opened in order for your body to have a reason to go down to the freezers downstairs to start using those energy stores.

Fasting and Metabolism

Won't My Metabolism Slow Down?

The very first time I competed in bodybuilding way back in 2004, I had no clue what I was doing. I found a guy to coach me and that he did.

But the problem was that he had just put me on a cookie cutter, extreme approach, probably the same one that someone had put him on prior.

I remember ending that preparation phase eating 1600 calories per day, not one single 'cheat meal' in 4 months.

Well, there were a couple of problems with that…

I wound up gaining 35 pounds in the week after the show!

And, for the next decade, every time I started to try and eat normal amounts of food, let's say in the modest range for a guy my size, of 2800 calories, I would get fatter and gain weight.

Devon was never able to understand how this could be, nor could I. I realized that I had messed up my metabolism and the ironic thing was I would try to fix it by following the same advice, eat a lot of protein and eat often.

For a quick lesson in metabolism, your basal metabolic rate (BMR) is basically the amount of energy your body needs to run all your bodily functions if you were to lay still, in a bed, all day. To figure this number out, simply take your body weight and multiply it by 10 in most situations.

That will put your pretty damn close to where your BMR is.

So, for maintenance calories in the traditional approach, if you add in daily activity and exercise and it should be quite a bit higher than your BMR in terms of maintaining weight. If I were to add those things in, I'd usually put it at your bodyweight multiplied by 14-16. (My BMR is roughly 2300 and if I was going to eat at maintenance calories it'd be 3200-3700).

For me, it would lead to predictable and consistent weight gain.

And of course, I would only make the issue worse every year, contest year or not, by 'dieting down' as the summer approached, each time, signaling my body to become more efficient on using the food fuel that made up my diet. If it became more efficient at utilizing each outside calorie that came in, it meant a calorie would go a long way and it would get used to using fewer calories, not more of them.

How does this impact you? Put simply, when you diet and follow a traditional plan, your body will continue to drop metabolic rate to roughly match what you are putting in, meanwhile, your main hunger hormone, ghrelin, will continue to rise and leptin levels (which are found in fat cells), will drop, meaning hunger continues to climb while metabolism continues to plummet.

Numerous studies have shown that over four days of continuous fasting, BMR does not drop! That means that without eating for 4 days, there are negative consequences to your metabolic rate.

And, are you ready for this, it actually increases by 12%!!!!

The contestants from the famous TV show, *The Biggest Loser*, have been studied pretty extensively. Over the short term, the average contestant loses 127 pounds during the first 6 months.

But the reason there is never a reunion show is because they ALL have gained the weight back and then some (I believe one contestant has somehow managed to keep it off, making that person an extreme outlier).

In fact, over those 6 months, the BMR of the contestants dropped on average, 789 calories per day!!!! This is what is known as 'starvation mode', ironically, actually 'starving' has the opposite effect!

To make matters worse, even after 6 years, the metabolic rate does not recover. This is exactly what I had experienced since my very first competition.

• • • • •

How Does My Metabolism Actually Increase?

I recall reading a book back in the early 2000's in which the author had all different types of diets aimed at helping one put on muscle mass.

I am talking daily intakes of up to 8,000 calories per day, which is something mere mortals simply cannot do.

Needless to say, there was some useful info in the book, but it wasn't practical on many levels.

Now think about this, when you are eating good, nutritious food and you want to gain weight, you can bump up 500 calories per day and not gain much at all. You can go up to 1,000 calories per day and not gain too much.

What will happen however is that your hunger will dramatically decrease and you will get disgusted just looking at food.

The exact opposite of what happens when we cut calories goes on here. Your metabolic rate goes up (but not in the way the experts would have you think) and your main hunger hormones go way down.

This is why I used to force feed myself by plugging my nose and rinsing each bite with water. Talk about completely ignoring your biofeedback!

So, your metabolism goes up in this instance through something known as NEAT, which stands for non-exercise activity thermogenesis; which is a fancy way of saying the physical activity you do on a daily basis besides any actual workout.

Your basal metabolic rate, which I spoke about earlier, has the capacity to shift up or down 40%!

But in both of the instances, cutting calories or here, as in raising calories, you are still playing the calorie game. Our metabolism is basically the energy needed to keep the cells in our body alive while maintaining a temperature of roughly 98.6 degrees, which requires energy.

So, the long awaited answer to the question of how your metabolism can actually increase while fasting.

Remember back when I said that the only reason I began fasting was because of my research showing me that fasting can actually increase blood flow to the stubborn fat cells?
Well, to reiterate a portion of that, your body must be able to mobilize fat stores, transport them to the muscles and then have the muscles perform the utilization phase.

According to research in Siim Land's book (*Metabolic Autophagy*), when 'fat burning increases so does the amount of Uncoupling Protein-3 in our muscles (UCP-3). As little as 15-hours of fasting enhances gene expression for UCP-3 by 5X!!!!'

What this means in layman terms is that our muscles are much more able to use our own body fat as fuel sources during a fast of as little as 16 hours!

Further, 'After the first 48-hours of a fast, metabolism increases by 3.6%! Even more, 4 days in, resting energy expenditure goes up 14%!'

Yup, instead of slowing down our metabolism, our body actually increases it.

Now, here's another cool thing about metabolism from Siim's book: fasting increases sirtuins. 'Sirtuins regulate fat and glucose metabolism in response to physiological changes in energy levels; they are a crucial determinant of energy homeostasis.

There are 3 different kinds of sirtuins. SIRT 1 regulates mitochondrial growth. Mitochondria are the powerhouses of the cells; they are where energy production occurs.

'Suppression of SIRT 2 restricts fatty acid metabolism, reduces mitochondrial activity and promotes obesity'. And SIRT 3 has to do with oxidative stress.

An increase in sirtuins leads to an increase in your cells ability to produce energy from its own internal resources!

But if you are not fasting and you are eating every few hours, then you don't get the bump in sirtuin activity.

There you have it. Next time someone tells you that you are going to go into starvation mode and that your metabolism will stall, pull out this page of the book and have them take a look. ☺

• • • • •

That Ties In Nicely to the 'Juice'

Back in 2008 when I first hired Scott Abel, guru of gurus, to coach me, he turned me onto sodium supplementation. (here's the article: https://www.t-nation.com/diet-fat-loss/sodium-your-secret-weapon).

At that time, that meant I was using pickles, sea salt and soy sauce, to get my sodium in. Sodium is a great performance enhancer and for those of you interested, it gives you a fantastic pump in the gym.

In fact, it was around that time that I was working on the side for a large supplement company and I started looking at their ingredients in their 'muscle building' line and all of them contained sodium phosphate.

Most people are highly deficient in sodium. It's another one of the lies that the mainstream has bought into, hook line and sinker.

When we are deficient in sodium, we go through something known as internal starvation. This is basically when cells aren't getting enough of the essential, life sustaining nutrient of sodium, which in turn leads to an increased insulin resistance.

Yes, low sodium will actually lead to this because we produce insulin in response to low sodium in an effort to hold onto it. Remember, insulin is a storage hormone.

When people begin to fast and complain of low energy, in my observation a majority of the time it is due to withdrawal and their mental state.

Recall that most of us have an unlimited supply of food already stored away on our body. However, if people do actually have low energy when they begin to fast, it is because they are too low in their electrolytes.

Being that people are already deficient in their electrolytes, combined with the practice of fasting in which the few electrolytes they were getting, their levels will drop even lower.

Meanwhile, every cell in your body still requires the action of sodium and potassium.

And they continue to excrete their electrolytes through urination etc.

Once you add in 'the juice' (it got its name from Cole Robinson's 'Snake Juice' and I give total credit to him for coming up with the ratios), you can literally fast for days and feel great and perform great!

• • • • •

But What About Feeding My Metabolism Every Few Hours?

This topic ties right into the myth of needing to have a morning breakfast because it supposedly will kick start your metabolism for the day.

Or the one that says you shouldn't eat too close to bed.

Going back to what I have said elsewhere in the book, you need to always keep the goal the goal. For most people, not all, but most, keeping their weight lower or dropping weight is of key importance for longevity.

This means that we once again have to give the body a reason to use its stored body fat as fuel. If we are eating every few hours to speed up our metabolism, we signal the body that there is no reason to tap into its reserves.

A few key points about this:

First, who do you think has been saying that we need to eat every few hours? I'll tell you who; the food industry and its sub-branches of supplements and the sub-branch of that- the world of bodybuilding and physique transformation. It's really quite simple once you trace the dollar trail.

Of course the food industry wants you to eat more often because eating more often or taking supplements more often will lead to you spending more.

Second, people have confused the hunger they feel while eating small frequent meals with a sped up metabolism. It's nothing of the sort. A few years back, I hired an old Coach to give me a kick start again and while he turned my head around and opened my mind and emptied my cup in regards to eating more of a whole-food, plant based diet, he also had me eating the old 5 times per day.

This was tough to fit in while fasting and quite frankly, a big pain in the butt. One of the first things I noticed is that over the first 2 weeks, my hunger once again became out of control. I was 'entraining' my body and the hormones to expect food every few hours. Hunger does not equal a faster metabolism.

Let us use an analogy of a car. Suppose once again that your car is more efficient at using fuel. That means it will use less of it, not more of it.

Now let's suppose that the hardware of the car is our body fat. But this car is pretty cool, because once it runs out of gas, it can convert some of the hardware to fuel to use as gas. The problem is, unless we run the gas tank dry, it will have no reason to start converting the hardware to fuel.

If you are constantly stopping to fill up your tank, you will never run it dry and despite cutting calories, you will never tap into your body fat. All the bad things about dieting will happen when you take this approach.

When calories are adjusted for and you take someone that has cut calories, and added in more exercise, vs. someone that has simply fasted, the fasted person always wins in terms of weight loss and what goes on with the hormones.

Every single time you 'fill up', you stimulate a release of insulin; which by the way will lead to insulin resistance over time, especially if you are overweight.

We want as little exposure to insulin as possible throughout the course of the day.

Now, about breakfast just in case you didn't connect on this point earlier. When we wake up, insulin should be low and cortisol should be high. We do not want to spike insulin first thing because if we do, we are sending the signal to drop cortisol shortly thereafter and to store nutrients.

Your body can either be in anabolic or catabolic mode, not both at the same time. Anabolic means growth, catabolic means breaking down.

Breakfast as we know it is not the most important meal of the day. Yes, some people that eat a healthy breakfast can be healthier than their counterparts but it really has nothing to do with the food and everything to do with starting out your day with a healthy habit, which will reinforce healthier habits later on in the day and you will build momentum.

Why not just have some salt water and do a short walk with some pushups mixed in?

• • • • •

"If I Fast, Won't My Body Start to Store Fat?"

The year was 1997 and I was hanging out with my good buddies, the guys that dove head first into the bodybuilding lifestyle with me.

I was sitting on a porch reading one of the muscle magazines of the day, learning about how this bodybuilder, first name, Vic, can't recall the last name, would consume 10,000 calories per day.

The guy was a monster and throughout the article he spoke of the constant need to feed the muscles.

I bought in and I made sure to pack snacks with me for school, hurry home after school and make some fish or eggs, washed down by a banana mass shake, which tasted like chalk and then the every other day or so trip to Burger King to get some triple patty burgers, which of course were loaded with saturated fat and protein.

Now, you may be wondering what this has to do with 'starvation mode'.

Well, it's two sides of the same coin really.

You have those, like I did, that think if they don't eat every few hours, their muscles will melt away.

Then you have those that think that if they don't constantly consume food, their body will think they are starving and will therefore store anything that comes in as body fat in case you run into a period of famine again.

Ha! It's pretty bad that we have been led to believe that famine is going more than a few hours without food.

Starvation mode—a term that is often spewed out by the fake fitness experts—can actually only be 'triggered' by eating.

Yup, you heard me right. Eating small frequent meals has been taught by damn near everyone.

There was a study done around WW1 or two, if I am not mistaken, the Minnesota starvation study, in which they fed men, a drastically reduced amount of food, but they stayed in the 'fed' state because they never actually went more than a half day without food.

By the end of the study, these men were emaciated, looked sick and were malnourished on nearly every front. That occurred from cutting calories drastically.

Listen, your body has so many stored nutrients within its own fat stores that you could fast for weeks on end, as long as you are drinking the 'juice' (see below) and not be starved of nutrients. Yet, when we are constantly relying on an outside food source for energy and nutrients, we don't release what is stored within us.

If you connect the dots, then you can see that starvation mode is caused by your typical eat less, move more diet.

Fasting is a different road altogether my friend.

Fasting and Exercise

Can I Work Out on a Fast?

One of the most common questions that I receive about fasting is whether or not you can work out while fasting.

The simple answer is YES!

Now, depending on how long of a fast you are talking about, you may want to change your type of workout.

What I mean by this is that if you are talking about 48+ hours, then you may want to make those workouts more of a traditional aerobic workout.

But for most intents and purposes, when people ask me this, they are referring to eating one meal per day or even fasting for as few as 16 hours.

The human body is designed to undergo physical exertion in a fasted state.

• • • • •

Fasting and Your Muscles

Back in 2007, at the peak of my competition days, I won one of the two shows that I competed in, the South Jersey.

Interestingly enough, I got prepared for that show without having one single protein shake. Yup, you read that correctly.

It was one of the many times that I experimented to see real-world results on myself. Now, although this isn't directly related to longer fasting, it showed me that I could get ripped and stay muscular without ingesting protein shake after protein shake and eating a bunch of animal meat. One of the major concerns that people bring to me is that they are fearful of losing muscle or not being able to gain muscle while fasting.

Let me address the issue of the fear of losing muscle first.

Remember how I said that everything our body and brains do is done with survival as the 'main thing'? Well, go back thousands of years, just imagine, you were to wake up in the winter one morning and animals were scarce and plants were mostly dead or 'sleeping'.

This would obviously mean that food would have been hard to come by. Which meant you would have had to go out and hunt and search for it, sometimes for days. I don't think anyone can really debate this logic.

Well, your brain, which sends the messages to your body, came up with great ways to deal with this.

The first thing has to do with movement. If we received the message when we were trying to gather food for actual survival that we didn't like to walk for miles and actually 'get after it', we would have thrown in the towel and our chances for survival would have gone down significantly.

This means that movement and exercise make us feel good. There are certain growth factors and hormones that can only cross the blood-brain barrier via physical movement.

Physical movement is literally the quickest route to make us feel good and if you feel good, you are more likely to stick with your plan.

This ties into a quick point on exercise. It is great for brain health, which is the most important thing about it in my opinion and it is great for overall vascular health/blood flow and gaining strength and building muscle.

But, I'll be the first one to tell you that exercise is damn near useless for weight loss. Yes, you read that right.

Ok, the second thing that is pretty awesome that our body does when it goes for a period of time without food is that it increases growth hormone dramatically (2000-3000%!) which is great for mobilizing fat stores and preserving muscle.

And in studies on overweight men, fasting has been shown to increase luteinizing hormone (LH) by up to 67%!!! LH is the precursor for testosterone production.

In another study, fasting as long as 72 hours (regardless of whether the subjects were exercising) did not cause an increase in breakdown of muscle nor did it slow down muscle protein synthesis (the building of muscle)!!!

This means that not only is fasting very muscle preserving, but if set up right, it could actually help you build muscle easier!!!

And something I knew from my years of learning and being coached while bodybuilding was that the more insulin sensitive a person is, the easier it is for them to put on muscle. One of the main things fasting will do is make you more insulin sensitive and on the flip side, if you are overweight, it will help to heal your insulin resistance.

• • • • •

The Energy Edge

Any good plan should enhance energy and give you the edge. In my humble but accurate opinion, any good eating plan should give you more energy (the king of biofeedback) and give you the edge.

Energy speaks for itself, but what is this 'edge' I speak of?

The edge is a bit of grit, a bit of toughness, a bit of discomfort, all mixed together.

We've all experienced the edge when doing traditional diets—that feeling of excitement when you start out and that boost of stress hormones that helps us make it through the first couple of weeks. Only to have it flee once willpower is burned through.

When I did my first 48-hour fast, I remember thinking about how I was building mental muscle and how it was making me tougher.

It's all about how you frame it with fasting, but you also will come to know that after the first month or so of fasting, willpower is a non-issue. Portion control isn't the name of this game: a little bit of this, a little bit of that, nope. Feasting is what it's all about.

By mixing your finite resource of willpower with the way you are setting up your hunger hormones to rise with a regular diet, you have doomed yourself to failure. Remember, with fasting, the opposite effect happens; hunger becomes less and less over time.

Whether you decide to practice fasting or not, remember, any good plan should give you energy and the edge and it should be sustainable forever in some form or another.

Fasting and Hormones

The main effect we are trying to have when it comes to fasting as far as our health has to do with what is going on with our hormones.

With this, you also must keep in mind that food is a drug.

A drug is anything that affects the internal, biochemical and hormonal environment of your body. Food fits the bill.

One of the useful things that I learned when I was getting certified in Poliquin's level 2 BioSignature course (not the one where he berated me, it was the next level a few years later) was that 3 main hormones: cortisol, estrogen and insulin were the drivers.

The theory is that they have a trickle-down effect with all the other hormones in the body.

Now, out of those 3, the one that we have the most control over is insulin. Insulin is a master storage hormone, also known as the most anabolic of the hormones.

Anabolic equals growth.

Insulin, for the most part, is raised when we eat food. Some foods will raise it more than others, but know that if insulin is elevated, weight loss is damn near impossible because of the 'storage' message that it sends the body.

Poliquin also taught me about the 'fisching effect', which states that cortisol and insulin have an opposing effect on one another.

This means that if we spike insulin, cortisol will drop a short time later. When I first began fasting back in 2014, it made perfect sense to me because of what I knew about the hormones of the human body.

(Mind Map) The most stressful time of the day for the human body is when we wake up. Be clear that I am speaking in terms of a normal functioning body and what goes on with the hormones.

We are going from an unconscious state (sleeping) to a conscious state. Nowadays, we tend to wake up in safe and sound beds with protection via the homes we live in.

But you have to remember how the human body evolved and keep in mind that everything our brain dictates to us has to do with survival first and foremost.

Cortisol should begin to rise a few hours before waking and then peak when it normally wakes up naturally.

Cortisol is an alertness hormone, which makes sense given that we are going from a sleeping state to a wakeful state; one in which we would have to 'gather our bearings, located any possible threats, scan the environment and then begin prepping whatever need to be prepped to ensure our survival for that day'.

Stay with me here.

On a basic level, if we allow cortisol to continue to rise after waking, some hours later, growth hormone will continue to climb. GH is a fantastic hormone for what it does with keeping our body and brain young and it is profoundly fat mobilizing.

In fact, I once learned that GH produced internally (rather than using a prescription) was 8X more powerful on the body.

We want cortisol to do its job in the AM hours, it's hardwired into us.

Yet, if we are like so many other sheep that are following the herd off the cliff, we were taught to eat breakfast first thing in the day because breakfast is the 'most important meal of the day'. It kick starts your metabolism and on and on.

Well, eating breakfast will raise insulin levels which will have the exact opposite effect on what we want our hormones to do at that time of the day.

Most people will report being hungry and tired an hour or two after eating their typical breakfast of refined carbohydrates (bagel, cereal, muffin, pastry, etc.). And they would be correct because that is exactly the messaging they are sending to their body!

In all the years I have been Coaching people, I often ask people about their eating habits and if they are hungry at breakfast. I can count on one hand the people that report that they are hungry at breakfast, most people just eat it out of habit because that's what they've been taught to do.

To simplify, fasting allows cortisol to stay elevated, GH to remain elevated and keeps insulin levels lower. If insulin is constantly low, glucagon, the other hormone that regulates blood sugar, will be elevated, which will lead to more weight loss.

Fasting for Women

When I first began to study and implement fasting, I was wrongly led to believe that it worked differently for women.

I had read that because of hormonal differences, women shouldn't fast as long. Well, what I have found to be true is actually the exact opposite.

Women, more so than men, have often tried and failed/suffered through numerous dieting experiences. It is not uncommon to find women that are eating at such a caloric deficit that it almost seems impossible to believe.

I used to think they were lying when they would report to me what they were eating, yet they weren't losing weight.

And it seemed to get worse the closer they got to menopause, since estrogen happens to increase a hormone called lipoprotein lipase (LPL), which helps us to use fat more as an energy source and makes us less likely to store fat as an energy source.

Anyhow, if you are playing the calorie game, you will know from what I said already that it will not work and never has worked for more than a short period of time. The little benefit that you got from cutting calories is short-lived, and eventually you realize there is nowhere else to go but up, which is usually what happens (in terms of weight gain).

So, as women age, more so than men, they are already fighting an uphill battle with weight gain and adding to the mix insulin from eating and it's damn near impossible for them to lose weight, even while cutting calories (that was never the problem!). Insulin plus lower levels of estrogen in a woman makes it incredibly more difficult to get any weight off.

Circling back, what I have found is that women do much better even more so than men when they start implementing longer periods of fasting, such as 48-hour fasts and the like.

We had 2 women recently that had struggled to get back to a desired weight that they had been at recently.

Despite their best efforts, the scale simply would not budge.

Well, wouldn't you know, that once they began implementing the black version of the Panda Diet (one 48-hour fast per week and OMAD), the smashed through their plateaus, both losing 10 or so pounds fairly quickly and I am happy to report, they have kept it off, it was not a fly by night, cut carbs, lose some quick weight and then gain it back type of deal.

And remember the stubborn fat cells I spoke of earlier, the only way that I know of to increase blood flow to those areas (which you have to do if you want to be able to 'burn' them off, is too fast).

Fasting and Diabetes

Understanding Insulin

Way back when diabetes was discovered in the west, it was considered a disease of affluence because it was usually found in people that had access to a lot of frequent meals, rich foods, sugars and meats.

Dr. Jason Fung has done great work with his clinic and I reference one of his books, *The Diabetes Code*, a ton, when I am brushing up on my fasting knowledge.

Anyhow, I'd like to give you my two cents on type 2 diabetes (type 1 is a bit more complex). One gets type 2 diabetes because of insulin resistance.

The only way you develop insulin resistance is through inflammation and faulty eating patterns.

The way our bodies work is that they will build up a tolerance or resistance to anything that it is repeatedly exposed to.

Think of training with weights. The more you lift, the bigger and stronger your muscles have to become to handle that stress.

Well, when we are eating a ton of animal meats, refined carbohydrate sources and feeding our mouths frequently, we develop a resistance to insulin.

Your body releases insulin in response to blood glucose and insulin's job is to shuttle that sugar and nutrients to the cells for storage.

Over time, your body has to produce more and more insulin to do the same job. This is a very clear signal that the human body does not like eating the modern day diet; neither does it like complying with the modern day eating schedule.

Let me be very clear and concise in my opinion on type 2 diabetics. It works to 'cure' the disease, often fairly rapidly. Fasting heals insulin resistance so to speak.

Now, consult with your doctor of course to see how you can taper down on medications but know that insulin in the term of medication only makes the problem worse (leading to things such as blindness, amputations and neuropathy because of where it is helping the body story sugar) and makes you fatter.

Fasting will help us get rid of all the stored up sugar and it is not uncommon in a type 2 diabetic to have blood sugar actually go up when they first start fasting because their body is simply ridding itself of the sugar overload that has built up.

Dr. Fung cures people left and right with his fasting protocols, you should definitely check him out.

• • • • •

Insulin Resistance

I want to use strength training as an analogy here. What happens when we train with progressive resistance training?

Our muscles respond by becoming a bit bigger and stronger.

If we continue to train with progressive increasing resistance, we become bigger and stronger and so forth.

Your body has this response because it wants to be able to resist the heavier loads.

Your body becomes resistant to anything that it is exposed to in high doses.

We become insulin resistant when are constantly exposed to frequent feedings and are constantly eating refined foods.

Something that I have seen very few others talk about is this idea that when we set up an optimal internal environment by being more insulin sensitive is the concept of calorie partitioning.

Simply put, if you are more insulin sensitive, the calories you eat are less likely to be stored as body fat (without going too deep into this).

In a normal person eating a normal diet, let's say 50% of what they eat gets stored as fat and the rest goes to other systems of the body. In the genetically elite, more of the food goes to the muscle. These are the people that you can look at and envy because they are always muscular and lean, despite what they eat

This is something that I saw in full force while working with the Rutgers Football strength and conditioning program fresh out of college. Many of these guys went on to play in the NFL so we know they were the upper echelon of the gene pool.

Let me just say that a stick of butter and a cup of brown sugar in their oatmeal wasn't all that uncommon on a dude with an eight pack!

The last thing I will say about eating and putting on muscle is that if all else is spoken for, then it's really about the number of calories coming in for building new tissue rather than the amount of protein.

Here's a note though about putting on muscle, because people always love to ask these questions about diet and protein and packing on muscle: The key to putting on muscle is not diet. Nope.....

It's resistance training! You need to stress the hormonal and muscular system enough that your body gets the signal (those damn signals again, but remember all the signals of your body are brought about via hormones).

Training with weights or some form of resistance is the main foundation for putting on muscle.

After that, you need to make sure you are setting up the proper hormonal environment for when the building blocks aka food, comes into the system.

• • • • •

A Note on Bulletproof Coffee and the Like

For those of you that aren't familiar with bulletproof coffee, it's something that Dave Asprey created some years ago.

Dave is a cool guy, someone that I respect and someone that I actually interviewed for my very first book. At the time, people didn't really know who he was, but I did because I loved how he was getting after his passion.

Well, in short, bulletproof coffee is simply coffee with butter and MCT oil blended in. The idea is that you can have it and get your body to run off fat for fuel.

This goes in the same lane as KETO diets. If you get your body to run off fat as the preferred fuel source, then your body will burn more body fat.

You know what else will get you to burn more body fat? Fasting!

Someone had recently had a question for me on Facebook about using heavy whipping cream in their coffee since it was pure fat.

They assumed that it wouldn't spike insulin since it was pure fat and they were partly correct with that assumption, but what they didn't connect the dots on was that if your body was using that ingested fat source as fuel, it wouldn't be using their own body fat as fuel.

It makes perfect sense when you break it down and observe it, but it's this line of thought that so many fake fitness experts propagate that confuses people.

Just as in anything, you always need to go back to the goal. And remember that the goal is to keep the goal the goal.

Most people, not all, but most, begin on their fasting journey because of a desire to drop some bodyweight. Well, if that's the goal, then you have to remember that anything you ingest in terms of calories is going to negate that effect—regardless of whether it spikes your insulin or not. That is a big thing of what we are trying to do but by no means the only factor.

The easiest macronutrient for the body to convert to fat is yup, you guessed it, fat!!!

The goal is to keep the goal the goal!

Fasting and the Nervous System

Mind Mapping Principles for the CNS

Back in 2014, as I sat in the classroom learning Mind Map from Dax Moy, he further cemented my belief in fasting.

You see, a big part of Mind Mapping is knowing how the central nervous system (CNS) responds to life and your environment.

For our purposes, we want to focus on the autonomic nervous system, which has two branches if you will: the sympathetic nervous system and the parasympathetic nervous system.

As I mentioned earlier, the sympathetic nervous system is our 'alarm' branch of the nervous system. This is the state that most people spend nearly all their time in. This is your fight, flight or freeze reactions.

Some interesting things happen when we are stressed or under threat. The first thing is that blood sugar immediately rises because your stress and alertness hormones are jacked up.

Cortisol and adrenaline are released, causing us to figure out which of the 3 states is appropriate for the current situation. When these hormones are elevated, they trigger the sugar release. Then the sugar is released so that the body receives an immediate dose of quick energy out to our muscular limbs to prepare them for battle.

While that is going on, blood is shunted away from the stomach and gut. There is a really interesting book I read on the stress response some years ago (*Why Zebras Don't Get Ulcers*), in which they spoke of a Native American man back in the 1800's that had gotten into a life or death battle with a bear.

Unfortunately, he lost. But when his comrades were working on him, they noticed that his intestines/gut were nearly white, because of his blood rushing out from that area to be readily available to help him fight this beastly bear.

The reason that I am telling you this is because when we are under threat or in a stressful situation, the last thing we should be doing is eating. Yet, this is when most eat the wrong foods and at the wrong times.

Remember as I said earlier, cortisol can either be profoundly fat burning or profoundly fat storing, the latter when it is combined with insulin spikes (think about what your stress eating does).

This is why eating to the clock is so foolish in my humble but accurate opinion.

Just last night, I was giving a talk to a bunch of high-level, high school swimmers about nutrition. Now going into this talk, I know I have to meet the 'person' where they are at.

That being said, I didn't teach fasting to them.

Rather, when it got to the 'when to eat' portion of the lesson, I simply asked, 'Who eats breakfast in here?'

Only one of the 10 hands went up.

I asked the remaining 9 if they were hungry or not at that time and they to a T said no.

And I commended them for that, because I am sure their parents, teachers and various coaches tell them all the time that they need to eat breakfast because it's the most important meal of the day.

This gave me the doorway to tell them to listen to their body, if they aren't hungry, don't eat!

Now, counter that to the coffee shop I am in while I am writing this portion. A heavier set woman goes up to the counter, orders her espresso and scone.

Keep in mind that it wasn't even 8:30 AM yet.

As she is going back to sit with her friend, she said something to the effect of, 'I haven't eaten anything yet. I need to eat.'

I do not believe in judging others, although I am by no means perfect with this value. But I do believe in my reality math which is simply observing what others do and seeing if it aligns with what they want.

A quick little aside, I actually have a tattoo on my wrist that reads 'Philosia'. Nope, you ain't gonna find that word in the dictionary. It means the 'seer, the observer' and it means 'love'. To me it signifies bringing a non-judgment, loving eye to every situation.

Back to this lady with her scone. I can guarantee my left pinky that if you asked her if she wanted to lose weight, she would say YES!

But, she has been led down the fake fitness expert path of eating breakfast and eating to the clock. Thus, she needed to have her scone because 'she had to eat'.

By this point in the book, you should get a chuckle because it should be becoming more and more obvious that if you want to lose weight, simply fast, abstain from food for a period of time and allow your body to eat the food that's already on it, i.e.-your body fat.

• • • • •

Fasting and Brain Health

In 2014, when I began my fasting journey, I noticed that within the first few days of fasting, I seemed a little sharper and had a more positive outlook.

Now, keep in mind, I was in a completely unnatural state because of the shape I was trying to get into for my bodybuilding show.

Of course, I had nothing to prove this, but it made sense intuitively to me that fasting would benefit the brain.

Remember back when I said that fasting really went to work on your hormones?

Well, right out the gate, if we continue to allow our morning dose of cortisol to rise, it will bring along its friend adrenaline.

These two hormones are the main reason most people want their coffee in the morning.

Both hormones make us alert and are positive mood boosters.

I wish I was still able to physically feel the effects of coffee but I cannot.

You see, since my very first bodybuilding competition in 2004, I would use it strategically.

I'd only have it 2 days per week. I knew that the fat burning effects of it would be much more pronounced if I only used it sparingly.

It's funny; I distinctly remember that during that first show prep, it was Thursdays and Sundays. On those two days of the week, I would get up at 4 AM, make an entire pot of coffee, consume the entire thing over the course of the next 75 minutes or so while listening to some of my favorite tunes.

By the way, the reason I remember that so vividly is because of something known as Hebb's Law, which is a basic Mind Map tenet.

This Hebb's Law basically states that what gets fired together gets wired together. When you think back about your favorite songs, you can instantly feel the emotions you felt way back when it became wired into your brain as a favorite song of yours.

Music is a very powerful way to change your state and to bring back memories.

Now, think about how Hebb's Law is going to be at work when you start your fasting journey.

It doesn't just work with music.

The big thing that comes to mind for me right away is the typical American breakfast. For so many, people have been taught and told for their entire life that breakfast is the most important meal of the day and that eating breakfast gets their metabolism going and on and on.

The morning time has literally been wired in people's brains as a time for feeding and eating, so just keep an eye out for that and other associations (I told you Mind Map is everywhere!).

Back to the powerful and stimulating effects of cortisol and adrenaline.

They both are fantastic at freeing up fat stores to be used as energy in the absence of insulin; which is why it has always been taught in bodybuilding to do fasted morning cardio with a nice dose of caffeine/stimulants beforehand.

Now, along with the rise in cortisol comes growth hormone and other endorphins, which are great for your brain.

Lastly BDNF will rise during fasting, which is like fertilizer for your brain. I used to think through my readings that the only way to increase this growth factor was through physical movement but not so, fasting will raise it as well.

BDNF helps you to literally grow new brain cells and synapses! And in Siim Land's book, he cites research showing that BDNF can literally increase by 50-400%!!

Here is a quick bullet point list of the positive effects of BDNF:

- It contributes positively toward memory, learning and thinking
- It supports survival of existing neurons
- It encourages growth of new neurons and synapses through neurogenesis
- It has anti-depressant activity
- It decreases the risk of neuro-degenerative disease such as dementia and Alzheimer's

On that last point, remember that Alzheimer's is now being termed as type-3 diabetes; it is an issue of insulin resistance and inflammation.

As we have seen with everything so far, if your body never has a chance to take a break from insulin because you are always eating, then it does not have a chance to go through and clean up.

That ever-so important function of autophagy only happens in the absence of food.

Autophagy is the process of your body going through and eating damaged parts of cells. According to Siim's book (*Metabolic Autophagy*): "Autophagy is a metabolic process during which cells disassemble and remove their dysfunctional components."

It literally is derived from the Greek word *autophago* which means "eating of self."

Remember this, you are going to pay for your health now, or you are going to pay for it later.

If you pay for it now, it will cost you in terms of discipline.

If you pay for it later, it will cost you in terms of regret, not to mention your health, time and finances.

Fasting and Time Mastery

I am diligent with my time and energy management. So it may come as no surprise to you that one of the best things about fasting to me has nothing to do with appearance or health.

I love the time that it frees up for me.

Think about it for a second.

Time is the most valuable thing that we have. Once it's gone, it's gone forever.

Now, think about traditional diets and the food prep that goes into sticking with one of those plans. I know from having done it for years during my competition phase. I would spend hours upon hours each week getting the food ready. And most of the time it wasn't even food I enjoyed all that much!

In addition to that time, think about all the time you free up by not having to stop and eat every few hours. Not only is there the time to actually eat, which most people rush, so they mind as well actually skip the said meal (they are eating in the wrong state of their nervous system).

But, they don't realize how long it takes to regain productive momentum.

What do I mean by that?

Well, as I am sitting here writing this book, I have momentum. As soon as I stop for a period of time, it takes energy and focus to regain that momentum.

Allow me to use an analogy.

If I had you run 100 yards straight away and then run 100 yards, but broken up into 10 yard shuttles. In other words, you would run 10 yards and back, five times, which one would be harder?

The shuttle runs would be much harder because starting and stopping and then starting again is metabolically much more demanding that only having to start once. Your brain works the same way.

The less often we have to stop and eat, the more efficient and productive we can be and the more time we can devote to something else.

Fasting and Longevity

I am the first one to admit that when I first began fasting, I wasn't aware of any of the health benefits besides fat loss, nor did I care.

Well, it turns out that weight loss is just a great side effect in addition to the longevity that fasting promotes.

There have been studies for years showing that mice and rats that at fewer calories, lived longer.

However, when you dig a little deeper, you can see that while yes, they did eat less, but the more important thing was that they ate less often. Yup, they fasted!

So how does fasting put us in a better position to live longer, healthier lives?

As I have mentioned throughout, it promotes autophagy. This is when your body goes through and actually eats up and cleans up damaged and dead parts of cells.

Think of this as regular maintenance.

Second, it is great for brain function. My maternal grandparents are still alive and well at the age of 93. My friends can never get over how well they are doing and how coherent they are.

Well, the secret is, they have sharp brains and they keep their brains sharp by constant learning and connection.

However, fasting can add to that in terms of clearing out plaques that build up in your brain over time, which, by the way, are linked to dementia and Alzheimer's (another benefit of autophagy).

Add in a nice daily boost of your alertness hormones and growth hormone and your brain gets a powerful effect from fasting. I only repeat this because as the example with my grandparents shows, you are only as young as your brain health.

Lastly, and you won't hear many people talk about this; fasting helps us keep telomere length.

You can think of telomeres as the caps on your shoe laces. You know—the little plastic pieces. Telomeres protect the information in our DNA.

Telomeres get shorter each time a cell copies itself, but the important information stays intact.

Eventually telomeres get too short to do their job and either age or stop working entirely.

Simply put, the longer your telomeres, the younger you are, on the inside!

Fasting and Newcomers

When I first set out to write this book, I had the layperson in mind. I get so many questions from clients and staff about fasting that I literally decided to write the book on it (at least my take anyway).

And then, a funny thing started to happen. Other fitness pros in groups of mine started asking me advice about fasting and started looking at me as the go to source for fasting. There are even MDs that use me as a resource in that regard.

So where am I going with this? My point is that I believe you are either A) already fasting, B) thinking about getting started with fasting or C) are a fit pro that has clients that are interested in fasting.

The first step to getting people to convert to fasting is for them to 'buy in'. Think about life for a moment, all things start as a thought first and until that thought becomes all consuming, people usually don't take action.

With fasting, I never force it upon people. People take a religious-like approach to their food and diet.

Circle back to Mind Mapping, everything I do starts there. People need to be intrigued and want to do the action in order to form a habit around it.

Usually, there are key tells:

- People haven't gotten the results they want to get
- People are sick of the complexity of traditional diets
- People flat out ask about fasting

Here's a good Mind Map principle to keep in your back pocket: Don't give unwarranted advice. Yes, you have to be given permission to Coach. If someone doesn't ask you about fasting or how to get started on that path then don't offer it up.

Unwarranted advice is perceived in the brain as judgment and there is nothing more threatening to the mammal brain than judgment from another human being. Anyway, I digress (I love talking about Mind Mapping).

So let's assume that someone has bought into fasting. Depending on the circumstance, I'd say I have about 50% of our clients jump right into a 48-hour fast.

Why?! As I alluded to earlier, there is a lot of fear around fasting because people haven't experienced it yet. Your brain will be in 'threat' mode anytime it can't form a prediction and response pattern.

For me to tell them "it will be fine" is okay, but their experience that they will be fine is the ultimate king. Doing a 48-hour fast builds confidence right out the gate.

If people are ready for it, they will come over to your torch and decide to light their torch from yours. If they aren't ready for it, then just keep doing your thing, no matter or mind to them.

How to Begin a Fast

Long last, we arrive at the different protocols of the Panda Diet.

I've taken a long time to get to these conclusions and I have different lines of thought as to where an individual should start.

Once you decide, you must decide. Remember that a big part of the Panda Diet philosophy is there must be a clear divide; it's black or white, not gray.

Your brain will waste so much energy being stuck in that grey area otherwise known as indecisiveness and you will call your willpower into play if that's the path you take.

Making the decision is easy, once you have a strong enough 'why' behind your decision.

And allow me to bring up a few more 're-frames' for you again, because it is always more powerful to know how things work.

- Food is a drug. You are going to have different emotions that come up if you decide to try this approach. However, emotions are a terrible decision maker. Emotions and logic are formed in opposing parts of your brain. And it's the drug aspect of food that will pull you back into your emotions, which will try to talk you out of fasting.

- You have an unlimited fuel supply on your body, known as body fat. Fasting is the only true way to permanently 'eat that fat' and keep it off. A little hunger pangs here and there are good for you. We want to expose ourselves to hormesis, tolerable but lower levels of discomfort and stress. This makes the human body more resilient. When you feel 'hunger', know that it is just what fat loss feels like and that it is not by any means starvation.

- When you want to give in during those first few days because you feel that you need energy...know that the food you eat at the moment is actually costing you energy. Yes, eating takes a tremendous amount of energy to breakdown and partition the food stuff. The food you eat doesn't supply you actual 'energy' for a few hours. So that feeling that you need energy is really just you needing some type of comfort or stimulation from your food.

- You've been conditioned to think you need food every few hours. If you actually did need food every few hours, you wouldn't be here. Why? Because those genes that your family had wouldn't have survived if they actually did need to eat every few hours. You need to question where all this came from and hopefully after reading this, you will now be armed with the truth.

• • • • •

Different Fasting Protocols

When I was recently down in Florida for a mastermind with fellow gym owners, I was surprised by how many of them asked me if there would be a mentorship program for them.

I dug a little deeper and realized they wanted that because they didn't yet have the confidence to prescribe fasting to their clients.

And although you may think that everyone is into 'fasting' and it has gained a larger audience as of last, it is still a mystery to the mainstream.

Anyhow, as a part of that mentorship, I provide the most basic fasting protocols all the way up the 'Black Panda Diet' and then add-ons to that.

Depending on where your mind is at and what your goals are, you can decide between the protocols as needed. Just know that the longer you fast on a consistent basis, the more you amplify the effects and it is exponential.

Level 1

At this level, you can only eat fruit before noon? Why? Because fruit is digested mainly in the small intestine, which means your stomach gets a break. As far as your stomach is concerned it is 'fasting' since it isn't doing the heavy leg work of breaking down the fruit. Other than that, eat mainly a whole food, plant based diet.

This is the most basic and it is designed to really ease someone into this concept and way of living.

Level 2

At this level, you will be moving into the 16:8 protocol. This is the one that I did for years, with the occasional 24 hour fast. I have found through real world experience that this is the bare minimum one could do and hope to get benefits from.

This is a good one for people that want to put their toes in the water and get acclimated. You are most likely not going to see a big difference in body composition with this plan but you will start the habit and will get some of the benefits. With this plan, I recommend eating no more than 2x per day. The less often we eat, the better.

Level 3

At this level, you will be using what is known as the warrior protocol which is a 20:4 fast. This means that you have a 4 hour window in which to get your two meals in. One of these meals is going to be a little lighter than the other. You will start to get more of the body composition benefits at this level and will reap some more of the health benefits such as the positive shifts in hormones, reduced inflammation and you will become more insulin sensitive.

I have found throughout the years that a good amount of clients are very comfortable starting here because they usually go through their day and already do something like this. For others, it is really just a matter of cutting out breakfast since most people eat that out of habit and an emotional attachment to it, after being told for years that breakfast was the most important meal of the day.

Level 4

At this level, your life really starts to become simplified. This is where we enter the land of one meal a day, otherwise known as OMAD. It doesn't get much simpler than this, except when we get to the next level. ☺

This is great for people that are busy and that really want to get the weight off once and for all. You can place this meal whenever you'd like. If you were truly going by a circadian rhythm as to when the human body would like a bigger meal like this, you would have it around high noon, when the sun is at its peak.

However, for most people, they don't have an hour plus to sit down, midday, eat in a relaxed state and then relax for a little while afterwards. I prefer to eat my meal later at night, when I can relax for the day and chill out. I have always had my biggest meal shortly before bed, which is another thing the fake fitness experts will tell you not to do. I'd recommend testing the timing out. If you do it later at night, try to get a quick 10 minute walk in right afterwards, not a huge deal if you cannot do this but it is something I recommend.

For social reasons, since we do take them into account with the Panda Diet, most people find dinner the best time to eat their one meal.

Level 5

At this level you would begin to implement longer fasts. By longer, I am talking about 48-hour fasts or 72-hour fasts. This will depend on your goal and lifestyle. This is where the real magic of fasting happens. And it sounds much harder than it is.

If doing a 48-hour fast, I would recommend starting with one per week.

This is for people that want to gain quick confidence in their ability to fast. The best candidates for this plan would be people that have to lose 25+ pounds and menopausal/perimenopausal women, if we are speaking strictly in weight loss terms.

And that takes us nicely in the Black Panda Approach…

The Black Panda Diet

This is my own personal plan. This is the real, true Panda Diet as I created it. Based on your personal bio-feedback and check-ins, the following may be adjusted.

Sunday night-Tuesday night: 48-hour fast

Wednesday-Saturday: OMAD, one meal a day

Sunday (you can also pick another day if that works better than a Sunday): 'free' day, have whatever you want

*If you are going to have a few cocktails, on a non-free day, don't sweat it unless you think it's becoming an issue

*you are to drink the juice 2x daily (more if you want): in 32-40 oz. of water, do

- ¼-1/2 tsp. of pink sea salt
- ¼-1/2 tsp. of Lo-Salt or Nu-Salt (potassium chloride)
- ¼-1/2 tsp. of baking soda

*During the fast period you can also have coffee and tea. We are trying to form habits around this lifestyle.

What to eat: cut animal meat consumption to just 3x per week
Other than that, anything that grew from the ground/earth is fair game:

- Oats
- Fruit
- Potatoes of all kinds
- Quinoa
- Rice
- Beans
- Veggies of all kinds
- Grains if you do okay with them

I have found that placing your 48-hour fast after your last meal on Sunday does wonders for people. They enter the new week, primed and ready to rock and roll, which gives you an edge going into the week.

And, it fits nicely with most people's social lives as in everyday life. It is rare to have social functions on a Monday, which is really the only day that you aren't eating.

• • • • •

How to Use 48-Hour Fasts and 72-Hour Fasts

Depending on what your exact goals are, you can do multiple 48's per week and or a 48 and 72 each week.

This would be for those that have a serious amount of weight to lose in addition to those that are really into the pure health benefits of fasting, such as autophagy and the big increases in GH.

I recommend that if you don't have a lot of weight to lose, you do a 48 hour fast at least once per month and a 72-hour at least every quarter.

If you do have significant weight to lose, I would work towards doing at least two 48's per week. One very simple method for those that need to drop the el-bees is to use real time feedback on the scale.

For example, you feast, then fast for 48-72 hours, until you drop two pounds on the scale, at which point it would signal it's time for you to eat again that day and then repeat.

If you were 280 pounds, you wouldn't break your fast until it read 278. You would eat that day, then you wouldn't break your fast until it read 276 and so on. It's as simple as it gets and it depends on your mindset and the speed with which you want to get the weight off.

This also leads me to bringing up the point which I brought up earlier in the book; a proper way of eating should give you more energy and the edge.

You should be excited about your goals and your journey. Most ‘diets’ promise a claim of 5 pounds per month or a pound per week. Does that actually get anyone excited? I highly doubt it. If you have weight to lose, get that weight off ASAP!

As you can see, I do the 48-hour fast every single week. Some call this extreme, I call it dominating. ☺

In addition to the health benefits, the mental and spiritual components are a real thing.

How to Break a Fast

One of the most common questions that I get from clients is this, 'What do I break my fast with?'

For starters, you need to realize that you have just given your gut a nice break from having to constantly breakdown food into nutrients.

And being that you haven't had food for an extended period, the last thing you want to do is start stuffing it with junk.

I get the whole mindset that you have been programmed throughout the years to fill up on whatever you missed out on, but that is a mindset that we need to reprogram. Bingeing and feasting are two different things.

With the Panda Diet, one of the core philosophies is to take a mindful approach to your fasting and feasting periods.

When you feast on good, nutritious food, you are in control.

When you binge on junk food, you are out of control.

So, back to breaking your fast. I like to begin with a half cup or so of pure cranberry juice (bitter as heck) for iodine content, alongside a half a cucumber or so, chopped up and loaded with sea salt.

This gives me even more of the sodium and potassium that I am looking to get in throughout the day and is easy on my stomach.

From there, I have a cup of chicken stock, which is loaded with collagen and once again, very nurturing to our stomach lining and a big bowl of fruit.

Yes, you read that right and in fact, if there is one rule I like to have people adapt to their feasting a large percentage of the time, it's just this. Fruit first!

Fruit is digested in the small intestine, unlike most of the food that we eat, which is broken down in the stomach.

In fact, the very lowest level of fasting that I have prescribed is to eat nothing but fruit before noon and then we progress from there.

Fruit is loaded with nutrients and has a large degree of effect on our stretch flexors located in the stomach, which will signal us that we got enough down there. This is important, especially if you are still having issues with thinking you need to binge after breaking your fast.

Your Main Meal

After you've had your fruit, it's time for you to eat the main meal.

I want you to remember though that when you eat is far more important than what you eat. With that being said, I prefer to have a large majority of my food in the terms of what can be described as whole food, plant based.

This means anything that grew from the ground:

- Rice
- Potatoes
- Beans
- Lentils
- Quinoa
- Oats
- Fruits
- Veggiès
- And more!

I always prescribe about 70-80% as a visual to clients about how much of this should make up the majority of their food.

Do I want you to measure this stuff out? No, absolutely not, I want you to be mindful.

Yes, this means that most of the food you eat will be carbohydrate rich. Oh my! This is another thing in the Panda Diet protocol that goes against the grain.

The remainder of your food can come from animal protein. Yes, I prefer a diet that is largely carbohydrate based and I have seen great results for our clients and myself. Protein is more anabolic but this idea that we need gobs and gobs of animal protein is just simply not true.

This topic in and of itself is worthy of a whole book and in fact there have been some great books written about it. Here are a few great resources if you are interested in discovering the myths about animal protein:

- *Proteinaholic* by Garth Davis
- *Whole* by T. Colin Campbell
- *The Game Changers* documentary on Netflix

I tend to have animal protein nowadays only a few times per week, if that. And to keep it simple, you can have it on the days you hit the weights if it makes you feel better.

A typical dinner for me would include 2-3 potatoes (any kind), broccoli with some hummus, maybe some Dave's Killer Bread if you feel good on those types of grains and then I follow it up with about a cup and a half of oatmeal.

For the oatmeal, I subscribe to the overnight oats approach, except I make mine in the morning. I put a cup and a half (which will be way too much for most people just as an FYI) in a mason jar and fill it up with almond milk and maybe some frozen berries if we have them on hand.

Into the fridge it goes and now I have my dessert ready to go. I use stevia and cinnamon to flavor it and sometimes I mix in some nuts or peanut butter.

There you have it. That should give you a basic premise to work from.

I want you to be mindful of your digestion and smoothness of your bowel movements. When you start converting over to more plant based carbs and have plenty of sodium in your system, you should have nice, regular bowel movements, no strain, no pain. ☺

Digestion is one of the key signs of health.

• • • • •

How Much Should I Eat?

Once you fully adopt the Panda Diet lifestyle, you will invariably question how much you should be eating.

One the days when you are eating your one meal per day, if you stick with the recommended foods, you cannot overeat. I say this for two reasons.

First, eating predominantly a whole food, plant based diet, you will find that those foods take up a lot of space in your stomach, which will trigger the stretch receptors in your stomach. This is one of the signals that will tell you that you had enough.

Eating these types of foods means that you will be having a lot of bulk, a ton of micronutrients and a good amount of fiber. Your brain also has sensors that'll either trigger hunger or satiation based upon what micronutrients you are getting in your diet. If you are devoid of micronutrients such as zinc, magnesium, different salts and the like, your brain will pick up on that. This is something that is not often talked about.

Secondly, way back, when I used to do the Cycle Diet, which I reference earlier in the book, I found out quickly that you cannot get fat in a day. What I mean by this is that once you set up a great metabolic profile, you can handle a lot of food at once.

When I would be in supercompensation mode with the Cycle Diet, I would literally eat between 15-20K calories on my cheat day, no, that is not a typo.

And whatever you cannot handle will simply be burned off in the short term (food sweats as I like to call it) through your next workout or by passing through your system. Listen, your body can only absorb so much volume at one sitting, the rest of it will be passed through and excreted.

I have a very big appetite, let's say for simplicity sake that it is 3-4x that of the average man; and my measurements and biofeedback over the past year have proven to me that no matter how much I eat of these good foods, the scale responds favorably by staying the same (currently 11.7% BF as a reference) or goes down by simply adding in more fasting.

The Panda Diet was created to get you away from trying to quantify the natural and beautiful act of eating and enjoying food. If you feel the need to measure every morsel and count every macro then you are not ready for this transformative experience of the Panda Diet and micro fasting.

I was reading *Everything You Need to Know* recently and there was a quote that read, 'It takes sanity to think clearly, it takes insanity to think deeply.' Most people are insane in their approach to modern life.

I have a philosophy in life that whatever the majority of people are doing, I do the opposite. This has served me well in all areas but none better than in fitness and nutrition.

This Panda Diet was designed to be the death of traditional dieting and mainstream nutritional dogma. It will be bashed by the fake fitness experts, even though they see the high failure rate (damn near 100%) of their traditional plans—which make people fatter and more sluggish, and also creates more metabolic disease than it cures.

• • • • •

Bonus: Art of the Pig Out

Let me be clear that this isn't so much to do with fasting as it is a cool side piece, one that has been integral in my understanding of eating capacities and supercompensation modes. So, while it isn't' something that I incorporate full on in the Panda Diet, there is much to be learned from it as you will see.

Back in the spring of 2003, I approached one of my college professors in clinical nutrition with a theory I had been working on.

You see, I had been practicing 'cheat days' for the prior two years and continued to get leaner and leaner despite what the math would tell us based on calories in and calories out.

I rounded up what research I could get my hands on and set up an appointment with my professor, excited for the clarity he would be able to shine on my theory.

Lo and behold, I go in, hand him my theory and he says, 'I'm not too sure. I never heard of this and don't know of any research that supports it'.

As you can imagine, I was a little frustrated.

I knew that having bigger refeeds once per week was beneficial to me, but I didn't know exactly why.

I surmised that it somehow kept my metabolism from stalling out or dropping down too low.

Remember that your metabolism has the ability to downshift or up-regulate by 40%!

Back then, I was used to the traditional approach, cutting of carbs, cutting of calories and such, for as long as I could take it.

And having a 'cheat day' seemed to make it more bearable and gave me something to look forward to.

The next year, I competed in my very first bodybuilding show.

Through no fault of his own, the guy that was coaching me had been at about 1600 calories for 4 months straight.

When I say I was strict, I was strict! I didn't cheat one single time! And I felt like absolute crap.

Yet, it was during the few weeks after that contest that I was able to really notice the HUGE eating capacity I had. I had a bottomless pit.

And for the first couple of weeks, I didn't notice much negative besides being a little less defined than I was for my competition. But that was to be expected no matter what.

However, as weeks turned into months, I kept piling the weight on and I actually went into a pretty bad funk, which wasn't really about the weight gain, it was about my hyper focus on a singular goal.

Fast forward a couple of years, and a couple of contests later, and I had come across Scott Abel, the Coach that was finally able to explain the concept of cheat days through what he called his 'Cycle Diet'.

It was a dream come true for me. Diet my butt off and then have an all-out cheat day once per week (which would later progress to 1.5 day as I stayed within a certain shape and weight).

To achieve this state, I pretty much would diet at a big deficit, like I did for my bodybuilding shows, somewhere in the 1500-1700 calorie per day range, until my appetite continued to climb and biofeedback dictated that I needed to refeed.

Usually this was apparent in things such as increasing appetite and decreasing performance both in and outside the gym.
Once, I achieved that state, it was full go.

This meant I could unleash the beast and have my cheat day. On a normal cheat day, I would take in anywhere between 15,000-18,000 calories.

To a normal person, this seems like absolute insanity, and it was. But I loved every minute of it.

The only problem was that I would eat so much that I was pretty much comatose the entire day unless it was time for another round of food. Imagine those insulin spikes!

And then the next day, I would have a food-hangover (yes, as I have said over and over again, food is a drug).

My weight would usually bump up 12-13 pounds overnight. But that was okay. That was part of the feedback I was looking for.

If my weight increased 10+ pounds but went back to baseline by Wednesday, then I was in good shape to repeat it all again the next weekend.

There are some other legendary stories besides the Waffle House one that I mentioned at the very beginning, that's for sure!

So, how does this apply to the Panda Diet book?

Well, it shows the point, albeit on the extreme end, that the human body can handle a very large amount of food.

It also proves my point that you cannot get fat overnight or simply from one day of overeating.

On the flip side, it shows you that I have been to the extremes of dieting and you can be fully confident in my philosophy that it has been tested against the most advanced diets.

What I was actually programming my body to do with the cycle diet was to achieve a metabolic profile that happens in all normal dieting situations. I was cutting calories to the extreme, creating a pendulum effect.

This pendulum effect happens when you force the body to one extreme and you can predict that it will come back with equal and opposite force to the opposite direction.

An example would be when you go ‘low-carb’, you can be sure that you will wind up craving carbs, over-consuming carbs and lead yourself to believe that you are carb sensitive.

In the cycle diet example, I was doing what I have told you not to do with traditional diets. I was lowering metabolic rate, drastically increasing my hunger hormones and bam, HUGE cheat days!

Now, the problem with this approach is that it is not sustainable and most people can’t hop right back on their plan when that cheat day is done.

It is very sound in theory, but not in habit friendly science.

This was better than anything out there at the time and still would be what I was doing had I not created the Panda Diet. There were two reasons.

First, because I love to eat (which I get to do with my nighttime feast on the Panda).

Second, in traditional dieting, along with lowering of your metabolism, you will have a whole host of bad hormonal consequences such as hunger hormones going up, down regulation of your sympathetic nervous system which will cascade to things like having an impact on your reproductive system and immune system.

Again, stuff, I learned the hard way through dieting for multiple bodybuilding shows.

The takeaway is that you can allow yourself a ‘cheat day,’ off day, whatever you’d like to call it. It's good for the mind and the spirit.

And, the human body is designed to feast (although not to the extreme that I did in the cycle diet), not graze.

FAQ

Do you really think fasting is a good idea? Humans aren't meant to function without food. This was a serious question I received. I replied YES. Fasting is an excellent idea. I countered her point with some facts. Humans are meant to go for extended hours without food; that is the MAIN reason we store body fat. This whole idea that we need to eat every few hours is the root cause of the modern obesity epidemic. Fasting, in my humble, but accurate opinion, is the best thing you can do for your health besides getting adequate sleep.

But I heard that if I fast, I will go into starvation mode. Is that true?
No, that is one of biggest myths that abound. The ironic thing that what the fake fitness experts call 'starvation mode' is what happens when you follow their faulty advice of cutting calories to the extreme and upping your workout frequency too drastically. This creates a terrible metabolic profile. When your body is still reliant on outside food sources for your hourly energy, it will lower its basal metabolic rate to match what you are putting in. This is why you may get some quick weight loss that stalls out, the body is brilliant. Now add in excessive exercise and your body gets much more efficient at using body fat as fuel, not what you want. If it is efficient, you use less of it, not more of it. And your ability to store fat greatly increases when you follow the fake fitness advice of cut, cut, cut and workout more, more, more. Fasting has the opposite effect, hunger hormones go down and metabolism actually increases. Do not fall into the trap of using exercise for fat loss!

They say that once you have a fat cell, you have it for life, is that true?
Yes, once a fat cell is created, you have it. Now, its ability to store fat is pretty great, so it can expand in size. There is a lot of research that I learned about back in college that a fat cell can die away after 10 years, but for most people, for everyone that is dying, one is created. The goal then, is to shrink the fat cells. You can do this through fasting. As you may recall, the main reason that I began fasting is because it increases blood flow to stubborn fat cells, known as alpha receptors. Stage one of fat loss is mobilization. You can't mobilize if you can't get the blood into the area (part of what makes stubborn fat, well, stubborn). The second phase is transport. Fasting plays into this greatly. Be at peace because fasting will increase fat burning and blood flow to those areas and this means that you will shrink those fat cells.

What if I just want to lose fat around my belly?
There are a few points to note about this. Nothing, and I mean nothing, will help you to lose fat in and around the midsection like fasting. If you may recall from earlier in the book, the reason I began fasting was to lose the stubborn fat more efficiently for my bodybuilding shows back in 2014. For most people that have a problem with belly fat, you can be sure that there is a good amount of visceral fat (deep internal fat that surrounds the organs) and stubborn fat (which sits more subcutaneously; i.e., just below the skin). Fasting will increase blood flow to these areas which means the fat loss process can take place. However, there is no such thing as spot reducing. This means that your body typically will pull fat from certain other areas first before it gets to the areas, such as your belly fat, that you would want to see go first. But this isn't a bad thing, there's just an order for how this happens and the stubborn areas are usually last to go. You will see fat loss first in your face and chin area, followed by the limbs and then it typically works inward towards the trunk/gluteal area.

Why do my fingers and toes get cold when I fast longer?
This goes back to the reason that I started fasting in the first place. Fasting increases blood flow to areas like the midsection and stubborn fat, in order to mobilize and then transport that fat

to the working muscles. Well, if blood flow is increasing to those areas, it will slightly decrease to the extremities. I do find it much more bearable in these terms to do longer fasts when it is warm outside as I already have an issue with blood flow to my fingers. But each individual is different, just something to be aware of.

What is allowed during my fast? Can I chew gum and have things like crystal light?
During your fasting period, I recommend that you stick with black coffee, tea and the 'juice'. There are different studies that show you can and some that show you can't stimulate insulin secretion through artificial sweeteners. So, that is not the main point of withholding from those substances. I like people to stay away from them because it is what I call mental masturbation. If you need to have something sweet, you are more than likely experiencing the drug aspect of food and the symptoms of withdrawal. Once you have it down pat, then ok, here and there is fine, but for most, I like to start out strictly. As for gum, I don't recommend it unless you absolutely get in a bind, such as your breath stinks and you have a face to face meeting coming up. Gum stimulates the digestive system and will wreak havoc on your system.

What can I use as sauces and spices? I can't stick with anything that is too bland.
First off, remember that it is much more important when you eat rather than what you eat. Now, as far as spices, you can use anything you'd like. I personally prefer a lot of sea salt (can't get enough of that stuff!) As for sauces, I am not a chef so I would recommend stuff that is more natural based. If it has a bunch of sugar and fat in it, then save that for a cheat meal. For recipes, I recommend following Chef Charity Morgan. You can find her with a quick Google search. Socrates is quoted to have said that hunger is the best sauce. If you can't stick with a disciplined fasting focused lifestyle because of the lack of taste, then simply make your food taste better. No one ever said that your food should be bland. But if you find the need to take something healthy and drench it in candy masquerading as sauce, then it's an even clearer sign that you need to get fasting and allow the natural flavor of food return to your taste buds. I will tell you that when I was competing, and I got deep into contest prep, broccoli with mustard was like gold manna from heaven. Even nowadays, when I eat my nightly meal, I look forward to it with excitement and believe me, there is nothing exotic about it.

• • • • •

Just feast and let your body perform its beautiful function of storage, utilization and excretion.

Testimonials

Here's what other people have experienced on the Panda Diet:

• • • • •

I am 54 years old. When I came to Kyle to plan out my program to better health, he told me "Nutrition is the easy part." My reaction was, "I don't think so." Kyle was right on! He introduced me to the Panda Fasting Plan, and explained the purpose and benefits. I was still skeptical as I had never heard of this fasting process. I didn't think I could do it.

Into Week #2 of my Better Health Journey, I did get used to drinking the Panda juice, and doing the fast was not difficult. I did not feel hungry. I noticed a few changes in my body during the Fasting process. Almost immediately into the second week, the Arthritic joints in my fingers did not hurt anymore. The inflammation was gone, and so was the "stinging" which I felt every day. It had been getting worse, as I also took Tylenol or anti-inflammatory medicines almost daily. Since I have been on the Panda Fasting program, my joints continue to feel better and the inflammation has not come back!

The other changes I have experienced during the fasting process are increased energy, a Sinus infection clearing up without medicine, and the slight "whisping" sound I have always felt and heard in my chest is gone. I have "Chronic Sinusitis", with a pattern of reoccurring infections every 6-8 weeks religiously. The routine for treatment has always been antibiotics, and an inhaler for the slight wheezing in my chest.

Before starting my program, I had felt a sinus infection coming on. The usual symptoms: Headache, pressure on my face, congestion, and wheezing in my chest. Into Week #2, just the same as my Arthritis felt better, so did my Sinuses. I could feel the infection clearing up. Congestion was gone, so were the headaches, face pressure, and... amazingly, the "whisping" sound in my chest which I have ALWAYS had is gone! I can only attribute all of the above to the Panda Fasting. Thank you Kyle for guiding me on my journey to better health, and to feeling better than I have felt in over 20 years! I will continue.

—Linda

• • • • •

After watching my husband succeed in getting healthy and feeling like a totally different person, I decided to take on the Panda Diet myself. Before starting, I was the heaviest I had ever been, I was very sluggish all the time, I was not working out and I had no real limits as far as what I was eating. I felt so bad about myself and my health. I want to be around to see my kids graduate college, get married and have grandchildren, so I needed to get healthy.

I started right off the bat doing a 20:4 intermittent fast, along with one 48 hour (sometimes 2) fast per week. After 2 months, I can honestly say I feel much healthier, I am working out 4-5 times per week and I am down 25+ lbs. I have lost a significant amount of body fat, and built up my lean muscle mass. I am so thankful to have discovered this lifestyle change. The Panda Diet has changed my life and my path to being my healthiest self. I would recommend this to anyone who is looking to get healthy, lose weight, get stronger or just generally feel better about themselves.

—Tami Batten

• • • • •

Newell Strength and the Panda Diet have been a life changer for me. A little over a year ago, I was sluggish, overweight, and just not motivated. I was reluctant to change both mentally and physically. Once I joined Newell Strength, I was hooked. I began my journey with a goal to cut my body fat and weight. I became addicted to working out, thanks to the Newell Strength family. After many talks with Kyle, I attempted to try intermittent fasting. I wasn't sure I could do it initially. However, Kyle's words stuck in my head, "food is a drug".

I began with 18/6 and saw changes, quickly. The weight came off and the motivation increased. The best part for me was that I was able to still eat most of the things I ate prior. The diet does not mean you can't eat. After seeing such great results, I was hooked and began longer fasts—some even up to 52 hours. This has now become a new lifestyle for me. With this new lifestyle, I am maintaining my weight loss and my energy level is through the roof. It has even changed my mental state to see things in a different light and my mindset is completely different now. I am more positive than I have ever been, and that has helped me to have a better relationship with wife and my boys. I am grateful for the Panda Diet and how it has changed my life for the better.

—James Ghanim

• • • • •

The Panda Diet was exactly what I was looking for in terms of searching for a simple and sustainable solution for a clear direction to bettering my health. Since I began following the Panda Diet, in only 6 months I lost over 55 pounds of body fat, and reduced my body fat% by 14%. I regained energy, focus, confidence and the motivation to exercise regularly again. My blood work now shows the levels that were elevated, such as High Blood Pressure, Cholesterol, and A1C have become normal again. For the first time in years I am in control of my eating habits and they no longer control me. I would highly recommend the Panda Diet to anyone looking for a simple path to follow to improve your health.

—Craig Batten

• • • • •

I have struggled with my weight my entire life. I went from a chubby kid to a morbidly obese adult. Sure, I have tried to lose weight many times. I was told I was eating too much or I wasn't eating enough. I measured food and counted calories. Truthfully, that way of life is horrible. Who wants to walk around counting every morsel of food or never eating a carb again? Not me! These approaches do not work for most people. After years of this roller coaster I gave up completely. I desperately considered gastric bypass surgery. I heard about Kyle from my brother who insisted I give his plan and gym a try for 30 days. So I thought to myself, here we go. One more gym membership. One more person telling me to eat six times a day and work out for an unrealistic amount of time per week.

I met with Devin and Kyle Newell for a consultation. This consultation was different. It was a deep conversation about me and why I want to lose weight. It was about the deep inner thoughts you have that you never talk about. That discussion generated my goals. Kyle, Devin and the Newell coaches truly care about my success. I have been following Kyle's Panda Diet plan and small group work out sessions at least 4 times a week. I am down 28 lbs. in 4 months. I have a long way to go but that is ok because with the Panda Diet, Kyle, Devin, Newell Trainers and the other members I can do it. Anytime, I want to give up, I have a mind mapping session with Kyle and he provides the counseling I need to regain my focus. The Panda Diet is easy to follow. It is hard to describe in words but Kyle truly cares help people. He is there for all of us and his team follows his example.

—Sandy King

• • • • •

Five years ago, I was on the phone for my monthly business coaching call with Kyle when he had mentioned to me something about a new approach to eating he was starting to work with, intermittent fasting. He told me about the 16:8 method where you fast for 16 hours and then consume two meals in an eight hour window. This news rocked my world because for years I was one of those who was led to believe that the way to fat loss and a lean body was the high protein 5-7 meals a day plan. Week after week, I would cook chicken and broccoli in bulk and eat most of my meals out of Tupperware. That was no way to live and the idea of two bigger meals a day coming from one of the few sources (Kyle Newell) in the industry that have my absolute trust in sounded worth trying. So from that point on, I dove right into the 16:8 method where I would start eating at 1pm and finish my last meal somewhere around 9pm.

Over time, I started to notice some great trends, I was leaner without living out of Tupperware, my energy levels were higher, my productivity was better and my mood was boosted. I continued the 16:8 for a few years and then Kyle introduced me to the idea of just one meal a day which would be later named the Panda Diet. At first, I was apprehensive about diving right in so I started with one or two 23-hour-fasts a week until a few months ago when I finally committed to the one meal a approach sprinkled with a 48 hour fast once a month until recently when I bumped the 48 hour fast up to a weekly occurrence.

I am 41 years old and I am the leanest I have ever been on a daily basis excluding times where I was prepping for a body building show. I don't have to pack meals with me to get 5-7 meals in a day anymore. I rarely get sick. I get to eat a nice big meal with my wife at night without the idea of obsessing over what macros I am consuming. I enjoy my food. I don't have anxiety over what I should/shouldn't eat if I am on vacation or away from the safety of my meal prep. I enjoy my life more. The Panda Diet is a game changer.

—Drew Handwerk, Owner, Start Today Fitness, New Orleans

• • • • •

I can only hope this recommendation is found by a special someone looking for an absolute return on personal investment.

Having the pleasure of meeting Kyle Newell in 2013, I was drawn to his non-traditional path of positive thinking.

From proper mind-set and intermittent fasting to living a true life revolving around his family, the guy is nothing short of the real deal.

I became more involved with Kyle's help utilizing the "Panda Diet" three years ago after falling victim to a virus which laid me up in hospital with a bit of a scare.

Let me rewind a bit. I'm a gym owner, a weight room and fitness advocate, former collegiate athlete, former professional athlete (1 pro MMA fight but who's counting) what could I possibly have done better for my health?

PANDA DIET!!

It really doesn't matter where you are in your life, there's always ways to improve, and for me it was through fasting.

I could probably write a chapter about how Kyle's simplistic way of teaching helped change my perception toward food, OR how the Panda Diet created a massive domino effect of benefits within myself and hundreds if not thousands more, but this isn't about me. This is about you taking the leap toward an outstanding quality of life where the mind and body work together and you finally get the results you deserve.

Here's the thing, Kyle's passion and willingness to over deliver will speak volume as you read this book and become a fan.

A professional all across the board!

If this recommendation has tipped curiosity to take the next step, the only thing I ask in return is you pay this forward. There's someone out there, just like you and I, that'll benefit wholeheartedly from this book/program, and together we can slowly start providing beyond ourselves. .

—Brandon M. Kelly, CEO, Undisputed Strength Co.

Glossary

16:8 Protocol: Fasting for 16 hours and incorporating an 8-hour window to eat. I prefer people only have 2 meals during this eating window.

Bingeing: When you have ceased to control the way you eat and when you have cravings that. you 'need' to fill for a particular food group.

Black Panda Diet. This is the pinnacle of the Panda Diet. It includes a weekly 48-hour fast with one meal per day on the other days.

BDNF: Brain-derived neurotrophic factor; think of this as fertilizer for your brain.

BMR. Basal Metabolic Rate; this is the amount of food/calories your body needs when at rest to sustain bodily function. Think of lying in a hospital bed all day and the energy requirements to run your body. This does not include extra activity such as exercise.

Cheat Day. This is a planned off day or free day in which you eat what you want. Unless you are in supercompensation mode, the purpose of this day is to just give your mind a rest and to enjoy foods that aren't on your regular plan.

CNS. Central Nervous System.

Fasting. For our purposes this is abstaining from food for a specific amount of time.

FFE. Fake Fitness Experts. This includes a large portion of people in the fitness industry.

Fisching Effect. This was taught to me by Charles Poliquin. It represents the inverse relationship between insulin and cortisol.

GH. Growth Hormone, a naturally occurring hormone in the human body that helps us stay young and is great for maintaining muscle and burning body fat for energy.

GI. Gastrointestinal. This includes all the hardware from your mouth down to your rectum. Most people refer to this as the stomach and the intestines but realize that it includes more than that.

HCL. Hydrochloric Acid. This is one of the main digestive enzymes that we have and it is depleted by chronic stress.

HSL. Hormone Sensitive Lipase. This hormone is elevated or must be elevated for fat loss to occur. You can do this through elevating other hormones such as glucagon and epinephrine, both of which happen with fasting.

Keto. As I refer to it, it is when people diet by trying to get their body to run off of ketones. Most people confuse low carb with keto diets. Keto diets are incredibly difficult to carry out and are not needed. Keto diets are typically very low carb and very low protein.

LPL. Lipoprotein Lipase; found in fat cells, needs to be inhibited for fat loss to occur.

Mind Mapping. The neuroscience of habit formation.

NEAT. Non-exercise activity thermogenesis. This makes up the biggest part of your metabolism after your BMR. It includes all activity that is not directly exercise related.

OMAD. One mea per day.

Panda Diet. My philosophy of eating. Black and white, mindful approach to eating. Realizing that food is supposed to be enjoyed but one of the best ways to truly enjoy meals and food is to go without for a period of time.

Pendulum Effect. When you force the pendulum to go all the way one side, realize that your body will react with an equal and opposite response in a period of given time.

PSNS. Parasympathetic nervous system. The part of your nervous. System that regulates resting, digesting, recovering, sleeping and relaxing.

SIRT. Sirtuins; a family of protein enzymes involved in metabolic regulation.

SNS. Sympathetic nervous system. This is the part of your nervous system that activates freeze, flight and fight. This is the part of your nervous system that activates via stress and during your workouts.

Starvation Mode. When you lower your metabolism and increase your ability to store body fat. Most FFE's have this completely backwards and actually activate it by the faulty low carb, low calorie diets that they promote.

Supercompensation Mode. Your body's ability to store excess amounts of nutrients in the muscle cells. This is dictated typically by super low body fat levels and biofeedback.

Refeed. When your body literally needs an excess amount of food to keep the metabolism firing on all cylinders.

End Notes

References

Abel, Scott. *Sodium, Your Secret Weapon.* T-Nation, 2008. (https://www.t-nation.com/diet-fat-loss/sodium-your-secret-weapon)

Campbell, T. Colin, and Howard Jacobson. *Whole: Rethinking the Science of Nutrition*. Dallas, TX: BenBella Books, 2014.

Davis, Garth, and Howard Jacobson. *Proteinaholic: How Our Obsession With Meat Is Killing Us and What We Can Do About It*. New York, NY: HarperCollins, 2015.

Fung, Dr. Jason. *The Diabetes Code: Prevent and Reverse Type 2 Diabetes Naturally*. Vancouver: Greystone Books, 2018.

Land, Sim. *Metabolic Autophagy: Practice Intermittent Fasting and Resistance Training to Build Muscle and Promote Longevity*. 2018.

McDonald, Lyle. [The Ultimate Diet, 2.0, 2003.

Psihoyos, Louie, dir. *The Game Changers*. Netflix, 2018.

Sapolsky, Robert M. *Why Zebras Don't Get Ulcers: The Acclaimed Guide to Stress, Stress-Related Diseases, and Coping*. New York, NY: Henry Holt and Co., 2004.

David Icke, *Everything You Need to Know*. 2017.

ISBN

978-0-578-68737-7

Made in the USA
Middletown, DE
11 August 2020

15006822R10053